The Hospital Patient

A Guide for Family and Friends

♦ RILEY-HICKINGBOTHAM LIBRARY ♦
OUACHITA BAPTIST UNIVERSITY

The Hospital Patient

A Guide for Family and Friends

Kenneth France

New Day Publishers
Carlisle, Pennsylvania

Copyright © 1987 by Kenneth France.
All rights reserved.
No part of this book may be reproduced or transmitted in any form or by any means, electronic or mechanical, including photocopying, recording, or any information storage and retrieval system, without written permission from the publisher, except for brief quotations in critical reviews. Inquiries should be addressed to Permissions, New Day Publishers, P.O. Box 134, Carlisle, Pennsylvania 17013.

Printed in the United States of America

ISBN 0-940271-00-1

Library of Congress Catalog Card Number 86-63036

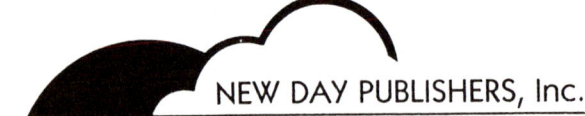

NEW DAY PUBLISHERS, Inc.

P.O. Box 134
Carlisle, Pennsylvania 17013
(717) 249-9557

"Visits are extremely important to the morale and well-being of the patient. Patients need to know that they have caring friends and family."

                O. K. France

                (my father—a veteran patient, a wise hospital visitor, and the person to whom this book is dedicated)

Contents

Preface ix

Acknowledgments xi

1. **Introduction** 1

2. **Offering Support** 6
   Providing Information 7
   Giving Gifts 10
   Helping With Tasks 12
   Offering Moral Support 15
   Assisting With Decision Making 23

3. **Choosing Your Response** 32
   Interrogation 35
   Reflection 39
   Sympathy 46
   Analysis 47
   Advice 49
   Reassurance 52
   When Communication Is Difficult 53

4. Hospital Visit Etiquette 56
Planning Before the Visit 57
Demonstrating Respect During the Visit 64
Staying an Appropriate Length of Time 70

5. The Patient's Medical Family 74
The Medical Family Tree 76
Interacting With the Staff 82

6. Special Considerations 89
Children 90
Patients in Intensive Care Units 103
Psychiatric Patients 109
Brain Injury and Stroke Patients 110
Terminal Patients 112
When a Patient Dies 121

7. Dealing With Hospital Crises 124
Hospitalization as a Crisis for the Patient 125
Hospitalization as a Crisis for Visitors 128
Patient Coping 135
Visitor Coping 135

Afterword 143

References 145

Index 155

Preface

Two years ago I was hospitalized for throat surgery. Although I had worked as a hospital psychologist, this was my first time to be an adult patient.

During my stay I had several visitors. I believe all of them intended to be helpful, but there was wide variation in their degree of success. Some effectively gave support, while others actually added to the stressfulness of the situation.

My experience as a patient brought home to me a visitor's great potential for good, and for ill. Consequently, two weeks after being discharged I began working on *The Hospital Patient*. Since then my efforts have included surveying hundreds of patients and visitors, contacting scores of nurses and physicians, talking with clergy and hospital administrators, and reviewing dozens of research reports. The result is a book that reflects the attitudes of visitors and patients, the opinions of health care professionals, current thinking within the scientific community, my own hospital experiences, and my 14 years of teaching helping and communication skills to lay persons.

The Hospital Patient contains practical guidance on how you can support a hospitalized individual in ways that will be helpful. I hope it will give you some new ideas, as well as reinforce many of your traditional efforts. My goal is to help you confidently and productively fulfill your role as a caring friend or family member of a hospital patient.

Acknowledgments

Thanks go to the patients, visitors, nurses, physicians, hospital administrators, and clergy who contributed their ideas to this book. Grateful acknowledgment goes to the individuals who reviewed the manuscript and supplied helpful criticism—Sharon DeVenney, Sue Shatto, Paul Herring, and (my wife) Mary France.

Cover design by Jill Brown

Typesetting by Charles W. Andrews

1

Introduction

You are not alone if you want to learn more about how to help a hospitalized person. Surveys reveal that friends and family members believe it is important to find out how they can help the patient. Lack of knowledge about what to do causes some visitors to feel uneasy and unsure of themselves. For instance, here are some typical comments.

- "I feel kind of awkward. I don't know what I can really do."
- "Visiting a patient for me is always a little scary....I'm never sure what to say."
- "I feel it is very important to visit a person who is hospitalized because it can help in the treatment of the patient. I feel visiting aids in the mental attitude of the patient. Although it is of such importance, I still feel uneasy visiting a patient...because I'm not sure of what to say."
- "I'm a little nervous about [visiting people who are hospitalized]. I'm afraid I will say the wrong thing."
- "The patient's life is 'on hold' while he's hospitalized, so there seems to be a communication barrier when normally there isn't. Honestly, most times I'd like to avoid hospital visits; a sense of obligation seems to draw me there."

The Hospital Patient

- "It is difficult to discuss their problems; it's hard to know what to say."
- The most negative part of visiting someone in the hospital is "seeing the person suffer...and not knowing exactly how to help."
- I feel "very nervous. I never know quite what to say."

Comments from patients also support the need for better informed friends and relatives. For example, both cancer patients and brain injury patients rate isolation and lack of meaningful social contact as the most troubling aspects of their hospitalizations.

Although friends and family members intend to be supportive and caring, sometimes there are awkward encounters that create discomfort for both visitors and patients. Rather than contributing to the person's well-being, some visits leave the patient feeling embarrassed or rejected.

Since there are good visits and bad visits, it is not surprising that research demonstrates the sheer amount or number of visitors has little relationship to patient progress. It's not the number of visitors that matters but what happens during the visits.

What is the difference between a helpful visit and an unhelpful one? Consider the following statements. Which ones do you believe are true with regard to supporting friends and loved ones in the hospital?

1. You should remain cheerful and avoid negative feelings.
2. It is appropriate to help with whatever tasks need doing.
3. When visiting friends, you should stay at least 30 minutes.
4. You should not touch patients.
5. Reassurance is the best response when a patient expresses uncertainty.
6. If you question a staff member's actions, a good comment to make to the individual is "Why are you doing that?"

7. When visiting a child, your departure should be inconspicuous.
8. A pencil is the best writing instrument for a patient in an intensive care unit.
9. Plans discussed with the patient should focus on what will happen after the hospitalization is over.
10. Most patients say the best part of being in the hospital is the support they receive from family and friends.

Answers for the questions are at the end of the chapter, but I will tell you now that the last statement is far from true. This book is intended to help you make the most of your hospital visits.

Published reports consistently demonstrate that patients cope better with health-related concerns when they receive helpful support from family and friends. Often visitors can do a great deal to ease the burdens associated with hospitalization. Research shows that even when patients are receiving the most sophisticated medical resources available, appropriate social support improves their medical prognoses and decreases mental distress.

Comments by patients and former patients also attest to the value of helpful family and friends.

- "The real importance is in the quality of the visit."
- Positive visits "made me feel better and helped to bring a speedier recovery."
- "Just knowing someone cares and can visit is the best medicine there is."
- "Knowing that people were concerned was a great help in my recovery."
- "Sometimes just knowing somebody cares when you're sick can be the best cure of all!"
- Positive visits help "the patient more than anyone can imagine."

But not all support is appropriate. Numerous studies demonstrate that family and friends can foster either adaptive or maladaptive patient behavior. As a hospital visitor, you are either part of the solution or part of the problem.

Visitors can contribute to patient difficulties in a number of ways. Research by others, as well as my own contact with patients, reveals a number of frequent complaints about visitors. The most common criticisms by patients are that visitors:

- overstay their welcome;
- excessively concentrate on the patient's condition;
- avoid discussion of the person's condition;
- give false reassurance;
- keep everything upbeat and exclude any opportunity for the honest sharing of concerns.

Visitors also can have a variety of positive effects on patient well-being. Patients report many beneficial aspects of having visitors; some frequently occurring opinions are that visitors:

- demonstrate caring and support;
- boost morale;
- provide contact with the outside world;
- break up the daily hospital routine;
- take away feelings of isolation.

Having read these two lists, some questions may come to mind.

How long should I stay when I visit? Friends and family staying too long is the most frequent criticism that patients have of their visitors.

How can my visit offer the opportunity for an honest exchange, while at the same time help to lift the person's spirits? One patient complaint is that visitors sometimes say one thing (such as "I'm sure everything will be all right") and communicate a very different nonverbal message (such as wearing a look of gloom or despair).

How much of the visit should concern the patient's condition? Some visitors concentrate on nothing but the patient's condition, while others avoid the topic.

How can I be helpful and provide support without threatening the patient's dignity and self-esteem? There are many ways to provide assistance while still respecting the person's needs for autonomy and self-control.

You are holding a book that addresses each of these questions. It is a guide on how to foster patient well-being.

Every hospitalization is unique, but there also are commonalities. *The Hospital Patient* presents typical experiences and describes techniques for coping with them.

The purpose of any technique is to give you confidence and to make you more effective in handling a particular situation. Having a plan in mind enhances your skills. But your effectiveness is heightened even more when you use techniques with flexibility and common sense. And that is the way the approaches described in this book are intended to be used.

As a friend or relative of a patient, there are several kinds of support you can provide. The next chapter takes a look at the possibilities.

(Answers to the true-false questions: all false.)

2

Offering Support

Patients give a variety of responses when asked to describe the most positive support provided by family and friends.

- "Getting news from the outside."
- "I liked the attention I got and the gifts they brought me."
- "They would help you with things that the nurses and aides were too busy to do."
- "They cracked a lot of jokes to cheer me up."
- "...knowing they were all praying for my recovery."
- "Being able to verbalize my feelings about the surgery."
- "Gave me support when I was afraid."

You can support your hospitalized friend or family member in any of these ways. The kinds of help you offer will depend upon your relationship with the person, as well as the patient's condition. Only offer support you feel comfortable providing.

This chapter discusses five ways of helping patients. It will assist you in choosing what support to offer, and it will help you decide how to best provide the assistance you give.

Providing Information

Many patients have told me how important it is to receive information about the world outside their hospital rooms. Here are some typical comments.

- "I would like [friends and family] to talk and sit with me to let me know what was going on."
- "I like when people talk about what you are missing at home/school and talk about what they are doing."
- Family members and friends "brought the world to my room."
- Friends and relatives "let me know what is going on outside the hospital."
- The best part of having visitors is "getting in touch with the outside world."

You can be a link to life outside the hospital, whatever your relationship to the patient. If you don't know the person well, you can talk about topics such as the weather, current news events, or sports. (It is best to stay away from heated political topics and controversial religious issues. You do not want to agitate the patient by starting an argument or by stirring up strong feelings.)

When you do know the patient well, there are a variety of additional topics that can be of interest to the person. For instance, if you both are members of an organization, the patient may be interested in knowing how things are going with the group. Examples you might talk about include work, school, church, sports teams, and service clubs.

Patients often enjoy hearing interesting news concerning mutual friends or events in the neighborhood. Some patients also want to hear about fictional events and characters. For example, if you both follow a daytime or evening television soap opera, the patient may enjoy talking about how things are progressing on the show.

When you know about ongoing events at the person's home, the patient is likely to be interested in receiving a status report. Common topics include how things are going with family members, how home maintenance responsibilities are being handled, and how pets are doing.

For patients who were unconscious for a time, there may be a need to know what went on while they were out. For example, an auto accident victim, who had been unconscious at the crash sight, told me that she was very interested in finding out how the wreck happened and who else was hurt, as well as the current status and location of the other victims. Should information the patient is requesting include very somber news, such as the death of another victim in this case, you will have to use your common sense about how much to tell the person. But unless you have an excellent reason for withholding information, I believe it is best to be honest with the patient.

Information on events inside the hospital often is of interest to patients. They frequently have questions about their condition and about how to deal with it. Sometimes you can provide support by telling the person how to get questions answered.

Illness, injury or the effects of treatment can cloud the thinking of a hospitalized individual. In such a state, the person may not ask questions that should be communicated to the staff. For instance, one patient recalled that his physician told him to drink water following surgery. After a half-a-day of having nothing but water, he began throwing up. When his wife visited and learned of his difficulty, she told him to ask the nurse what he should be drinking. The nurse said the vomiting probably was due to excessive water drinking and that ginger ale would be better for him. Soon after he made the switch from water to ginger ale the nausea subsided.

Providing such guidance is likely to be most important when the patient is having difficulty thinking clearly. At those times it can be very helpful to step in and recommend an appropriate resource. But I am not suggesting that you provide medical information.

All of us have home remedies for various health concerns, but these should never be given to a patient without staff approval. Many remedies, for instance chicken soup, have been found to have some genuine health benefits, and, at worst, most of these practices do no harm. But there are two kinds of situations in which the risks of a home remedy outweigh the benefits.

Home remedies that are in conflict with recommended medical procedures are likely to do the patient more harm than good. For instance, although chicken soup can be a good remedy, giving food to a patient who is scheduled for major surgery in two hours could lead to vomiting during the procedure and death by asphyxiation.

Other situations in which home remedies should be avoided are when the patient's condition is relatively unusual and when the reason for the person's symptoms has not yet been diagnosed. Continuing with the chicken soup example, if the patient is allergic to chicken soup, this tried and true folk medicine actually will make the person worse.

In addition to folk medicine, another source of medical opinions is your experience, or the experience of someone you know, with a situation similar to what the patient is facing. Maybe you had the same condition, you know someone who did, or you read about a similar case. You may be tempted to use this information to diagnose the patient's problem or to recommend treatment. Sometimes this kind of generalization is justified, especially if your experience is consistent with the patient's medical diagnosis and care. But there are other instances in which important differences exist between your experience and the present condition of the patient; unfortunately, those distinctions may not be obvious to you or to the patient. Overlooking such differences is the main danger in generalizing from limited personal experience.

Whether the information is correct or not, patients generally look askance at medical advice provided by friends and relatives. The person is much more likely to use the information if it comes from an individual whom the patient perceives to be an expert. So even if you think you know the answer, the patient is more likely to believe diagnosis and treatment information that comes from medical professionals. (Advice giving is discussed further in Chapter 3.)

Giving Gifts

There are many different kinds of gifts that patients appreciate.

- "It made me very pleased to receive so many cards and flowers. Many of the people visiting brought flowers or a small gift with them. The people I teach with had some of their classes in elementary school make cards and [they sent them to me] in a big enevelope. It lifted my spirits to read the cards the children colored and wrote messages on."
- "I'd like to play more games and have more books to read."
- "I would appreciate little things from home such as a book to read or magazines, cards made [by] my children, and a pretty flower arrangement....To be honest, I would be pleased to have anyone

bring some good home-baked cookies to me while I was in the hospital."
- "I'd want my friends and family to bring me things to read and keep me busy while they weren't there."
- A memorable gift was when "my grandson gave me some cookies that he made and told me what was in them and how they were mixed."

Keep the patient's condition in mind should you decide to bring a gift. For instance, don't take a box of chocolates to a person hospitalized for removal of a stomach ulcer or a book to a person who has had cataract surgery.

With the medical staff's approval, a permissible gift of food can be an excellent idea. It is not uncommon for hospitalized individuals to lose interest in eating. The patient's decreased appetite may be due to the hospital food, may result from the medical condition, or may be a combination of the two. Helping a patient regain an interest in food can be a valuable service offered by a friend or relative.

With prior approval from the attending physician, you might be able to bring your friend or relative a home-cooked meal or a take-out order from the person's favorite fast-food restaurant. Often such a gesture can help to rekindle the individual's appetite.

Several former patients told me that a gift of food was one of the highlights of their hospitalization. Homemade cookies seem to be a common favorite. Another person recalled enjoying some of her "mother's famous ice tea." But the food need not be homemade to be appreciated. One individual told me about the joy of eating "pizza!!" and another remembered the pleasure of having "real food from McDonalds."

Many patients also appreciate gifts that help them pass the time. A person who is able to read may enjoy a book, magazine or newspaper. Other popular items include games and puzzles.

Patients who were able to write have told me that they appreciated receiving writing supplies. If your friend or family member wants to write, you might consider giving note paper, envelopes and stamps.

Toiletry items may make a good present. For instance, one patient's most memorable gift was a bottle of perfume.

One of the best gifts I have encountered is a small cassette tape player with earphones. For the cost of a couple of hardback novels or a large flower arrangement, you can give a tape player and a couple of cassettes. (For a few dollars more you can buy a machine that also has a radio.) Knowing that the patient has a player, other visitors can add to the person's tape collection. In addition to music tapes, you also might consider giving the patient tapes of comedians you both like.

But what if the patient's room already is full of gifts? You may want to wait until the person is home before sending yours. One of the most memorable gifts I received following my recent surgery was a bunch of balloons—delivered to me the week after I left the hospital. The "pick-me-up" from such a posthospitalization gift can be worth the wait. (You also may want to consider visiting the person after discharge. Some patients feel abandoned if there are many visits at the hospital but few or none after they return home.)

Helping With Tasks

Hospitalized individuals often have difficulties carrying out normal duties. Consequently, the patient may appreciate your help with certain tasks.

- "I would like family and friends to help me with anything that I would not be able to do myself."

- "Friends and family should help me to do things if I need help."
- "I'd like my friends and family to get me anything I couldn't get for myself."
- I would like visitors to "help me out where needed."
- My husband told me "he would do the work when I got home, until I felt better."

You can help with tasks both inside and outside the hospital. Within the hospital, there are some kinds of task assistance that almost any visitor can provide. Common activities include getting ice and drinks (for a patient allowed to have them), reading get-well cards and notes to the person, and watering flowers that have been brought to the room.

Several patients have told me they appreciated family members helping them to and from the bathroom. Using a bedpan is difficult for many people, and often a patient would prefer to be assisted to the bathroom. With staff approval, the patient may appreciate your offer of such aid.

Some medical personnel believe that one of the most valuable roles for family and friends is helping the patient at mealtime. If the person does need assistance in eating, you may be able to provide a degree of support that might not be available otherwise. Small but much appreciated tasks can include taking off dish covers, inserting a straw in a glass, or cutting up meat and vegetables. If it is difficult for the patient to hold utensils, it may be appropriate for you to pick up a fork full of food and offer it to the person. (Some patients are too proud to ask for such assistance but gladly accept it when the help is provided in a matter-of-fact way.)

Also with staff approval, it may be appropriate for you to assist with tasks such as bathing and hair washing. Several former patients told me that they appreciated their mothers washing their hair while they were in the hospital.

If the patient declines your offer of assistance, you probably should accept the person's decision. You do not want to discourage or prevent a patient from accomplishing manageable tasks. Hospitalized individuals often see such oversolicitous behavior as forcing disability upon them.

Whether or not you help inside the hospital, the patient may appreciate assistance with outside tasks; this is very likely if the hospitalization is either lengthy or unexpected. For instance, I encountered one patient who had been hospitalized for a broken leg suffered in an auto accident. He told me that he appreciated a friend arranging "to take my possessions and vehicle home."

The sister of a woman hospitalized for four months helped with a number of tasks—among them her sister's Christmas shopping. "She would write down or tell me what to order; I would order it and pick it up for her. We then wrapped it together" in her room.

Other examples of outside task support include bringing the person's mail, checking on pets, taking care of household maintenance chores, providing child care and running errands. Your assistance with outside jobs can be especially appreciated, since being in the hospital makes it impossible for the patient to do many routine but necessary chores.

Even if the individual does not have an immediate need for assistance with such tasks, merely offering your services can help to ease the person's mind. The patient is likely to feel more secure knowing that you can be relied upon in time of need. Should assistance be required, the person knows that you can be counted on to help.

Whether or not the patient needs help with tasks, such aid may be appreciated by the immediate family. For instance, a patient's spouse may gratefully accept an offer to assist with child care, running errands or helping with household responsibilities.

Offering Moral Support

- I want friends and family "to give me moral support."
- "I feel it is extremely important [to visit people who are hospitalized] because patients tend to get bored and also they need moral support. When my mother was hospitalized for breast cancer, it was important for her to have visitors because she was very scared and depressed. When you give patients moral support they usually recover faster."
- "I think just telling stories about the past would cheer me up and help me get through the period."
- "One of my major complaints about visitors was the lack of conversation. It was difficult to get beyond the 'so how are you feeling' stage without discussing depresssing and touchy subjects. It would have been much easier if the visitors would have come with a conversation idea in mind."
- "I appreciated the people who were not too serious—who made me laugh."
- "Being able to talk to [family and friends] and knowing they were all praying for my recovery" was the most positive aspect of having visitors.
- I want visitors "to ask me how I am feeling."
- "I would like my family and friends to talk about things outside the hospital and [be] mildly concerned about what was happening to me, not needing all the gory details."

As you can see, moral support means different things to different people. But everyone agrees that moral support boosts the person's morale and self-esteem. There are a number of ways you can help to bring about these results.

Discussing pleasant times almost always is appreciated by patients. Reminiscing about fun activities you have had together may be enjoyable for both of you. In addition to looking back, you also may be able to look forward to the future and to activities you will share after the person is well again.

Joking and kidding around is appropriate with some patients. If you feel comfortable in this role, providing a good laugh can be an effective morale booster.

Humor can allow the release of pent-up emotions. If you are looking for a topic, try stories about people who buck the system.

Those in authority constantly are telling hospitalized patients what to do. Humor with authority figures as the butt of the joke can provide an outlet for expressing the loss of control that many patients feel. Jokes and stories that focus on characters who successfully outwit the system can provide a release for frustrations the patient may be harboring.

The humor should not focus on medical personnel, since you don't want to undermine a patient's trust in the staff. Any other authority system will suffice. A patient tired of being told what to do, still will be able to identify with the protagonist.

Since I am a college professor, I will give you an example from the academic setting. I heard the following story while doing my internship at the University of Florida's Shands Teaching Hospital.

At the end of the spring term, 200 students filed into a small auditorium to take their final exam in ornithology (the study of birds). As they entered the room, they saw a curious arrangement on the stage. There were ten objects with pillowcases over them; protruding at the bottom of each was a pair of bird

Offering Support

feet. The students surmised that each pillowcase covered a stuffed bird.

As they waited nervously for the professor to arrive, the students were abuzz about the purpose of the mysterious arrangement on the stage. When the instructor finally did enter the room, he announced that for the final exam the students were to identify each of the covered birds by studying its feet. There would be no other questions on the test. As a low rumble passed through the auditorium, one of the students at the front of the room stood up and addressed the professor in a loud and excited voice.

"You mean I've studied beaks and eyes, plumage and flight patterns, nesting habits and all that other stuff—and you expect me to identify these birds just by looking at their feet!!? Well, you know what your can do with your exam!!" In disgust he slammed his book on the desk and began to stomp out of the room.

"Wait a minute, young man," the somewhat befuddled professor called out. "I must know who you are. What is your name?"

The student turned swiftly, yanked his pants leg up to his knee and shouted "YOU GUESS!!"

This is one example of a story that pokes fun at authority. Patients are likely to enjoy similar tales that allow them to release their pent-up emotions.

But you should keep in mind two notes of caution about humor. First, laughter may be painful for some patients. One person hospitalized for an appendectomy had the following complaint about her visitors: "Sometimes they really made me laugh and that hurt like someone stabbed me." Ease off on the levity if it increases the person's discomfort, rather than decreasing it. Second, don't use humor as a way of avoiding the truth. For instance, death or terminal illness never should be the subject of a visitor's jokes.

Humor is one way of providing moral support. But more serious approaches also may be appreciated.

Prayer and scripture reading may be comforting to the patient. Although most often offered by clergy, some friends and family members include these activities in their visits. If you are one of those who wants to offer such support, the following paragraphs are intended for you.

The patient may appreciate hearing you read an inspirational passage. Your selection may come from recent services missed by the patient, from a denominational worship book, from a volume of poetry, or it may be a favorite of yours or of the patient.

For instance, one man visited a friend who was too ill to talk, so he read a psalm to her. Once during his reading she moaned as though she wanted to say something, and he paused. But she was silent again, so he continued with the passage. At the end of the psalm she looked at him and said "That was lovely"—the only words she spoke during his visit.

Just as a passage of scripture may be appreciated, prayer led by a visitor also may bring comfort and strength. Each person who prays has a usual style of prayer. Still, should you decide to pray with a patient, I would like you to consider four suggestions.

☐ Touch the patient as you pray (I have more to say about touch in Chapter 4).
☐ During your prayer, include a reminder that others are thinking about and praying for the patient.
☐ Be sure your prayer recognizes the patient's hopes and concerns.
☐ Keep your prayer brief and simple.

A prayer that is consistent with these recommendations is likely to be a source of comfort for a patient who prays with you. But not all prayers by visitors are comforting.

One person hospitalized after an automobile accident told me about a visitor who "prayed and in the prayer he said he was 'thankful that no one was injured.' If no one was injured, it's funny that I spent two weeks in the hospital. I resented his visit."

Should you offer a prayer, be sure to think about what you pray.

Uncertainty is one experience common to all hospitalized patients. No matter what the patient's condition, the person is likely to have doubts. For example: How serious is my situation? What does this new symptom mean? Will the procedure be successful? What will recovery be like?

It is natural to want to decrease the patient's uncertainty. And, in fact, research shows that patients often turn to friends and relatives as a way of decreasing their distress. Since your response to the patient's doubts can have a profound impact upon the person, you should carefully consider any efforts intended to lessen the individual's uncertainty.

When we find ourselves facing an ambiguous situation, we often seek opinions from others in order to feel more certain about what is happening. Social psychologists call this phenomenon *social comparison*, and a patient seeking your views is one example of this common kind of interaction.

Just as patients frequently seek out others' opinions, it also is common for friends and relatives to offer their views about diagnosis and treatment. This willingness on the part of some visitors to offer their views has implications for those who choose not to offer opinions about diagnosis and treatment. If others have offered their views, the patient may interpret another person's failure to do so as a lack of concern or as an indication that the patient's condition is much worse than previously indicated. So, even declining to give an opinion can have important effects on the person.

Why would a visitor decide not to give an opinion about the patient's condition? You probably can think of many good reasons. For example, you want the patient to get better, but if you think the prognosis is poor, you justifiably may not want to share your belief with the patient. Or you may not know enough about the patient's condition to have an opinion about diagnosis and care. Unfortunately, a reluctance to discuss the patient's situation can cause the person a good deal of apprehension and anxiety. Consequently, avoiding discussion of the person's condition may turn out to be more stressful than anything you might say.

So what should you do when faced with the patient's uncertainty? There are pros and cons associated with avoiding illness-related discussion, advocating folk medicine procedures and generalizing from your own experience. An alternative is to offer the patient a positive relationship. This is an excellent response to the uncertainty commonly experienced by hospitalized individuals.

A positive relationship with a patient enhances your visit, no matter what activities you share together. The offer of such a relationship can be an important kind of moral support and a vital source of strength for the individual.

Being hospitalized means the person needs help in coping with a health problem. Such an event can cause doubt regarding the wisdom of past behaviors or concern about one's ability to handle future difficulties. The person may feel less able to fulfill traditional roles such as father, mother, son, daughter, neighbor, friend or worker. Any of these threats can decrease the patient's self-esteem.

An appropriate way of helping a person deal with self-doubt and uncertainty is to provide an opportunity for the open expression of feelings and concerns. This kind of support is best offered by a person in whom the patient is willing to confide. You can be such a confidant if the patient trusts you and receives respect and understanding from you. When trust, respect and understanding characterize your interaction, you have a positive relationship, whatever your role in the patient's life.

To be trusted, the person needs to perceive that you mean what you say—that you are not putting up some kind of facade. Being genuine in this way does not mean that you must share everything you are thinking, but it does require that you be honest in what you say.

Unfortunately, friends and family members commonly believe they must remain cheerful and optimistic with patients. But pretending everything is fine can make one very uncomfortable. For instance, one visitor told me "I feel sort of awkward standing around the bed, trying to be cheery." And such an attitude of unrealistic optimism merely demonstrates to the patient that the visitor cannot be trusted to be honest. Encountering false optimism simply becomes an added stress on the patient.

If you respect the patient, you care for the person and want things to work out for the best, but you do not try to impose your values and beliefs. Respect means you recognize the patient's right to opinions and attitudes that may be different from your own. Demonstrating continued caring and respect is reassuring to the patient, especially if the hospitalization is associated with threats to one's usual life style.

Sometimes it is hard not to argue with the patient about

beliefs when you are sure the person is wrong. For example, research on accident victims who are paralyzed and on rape victims shows that members of both of these patient groups often blame themselves for their injuries. The natural reaction of many friends and relatives is to deny the validity of this self-blame. Whether it is accurate or not, blaming themselves for their predicament actually may be therapeutic. Being responsible for what has happened in the past implies that the person also can control what happens in the future. Seen in this light, self-blame can enhance recovery if it motivates the person toward productive, health-promoting behavior. So even though you may disagree with the patient, it often is best to be accepting and nonjudgmental.

Many visitors also have a difficult time communicating understanding to patients. For example, in one study of breast cancer patients, 72% of the women believed others misunderstood them. These data are consistent with the findings of another study in which healthy individuals commonly believed that it was harmful for ill persons to discuss their thoughts and feelings. To the contrary, what that study found to be harmful was the avoidance of open communication by friends and relatives. Rather than agreeing with "sweeping things under the rug," patients were disturbed and confused by such avoidance.

An excellent way to demonstrate understanding is to summarize the essential thoughts and feelings that the person has communicated to you. This kind of response is called reflection, and it is discussed in the next chapter.

You may be a relative of the patient or a friend. You may have a long-standing relationship or a relatively brief one. But what is most important in offering a positive relationship is whether you are seen as a person who can be trusted, who offers respect, and who demonstrates understanding. If these three elements characterize your relationship, you will be providing valuable moral support because the patient will feel comfortable confiding in you.

Respect, understanding and honesty are the key ingredients in a positive relationship. When a patient perceives those traits in you, feelings of enhanced self-worth are likely to follow. And by demonstrating your continued caring, you will have reinforced the patient's sense of belonging. In fact, of all the ways you can help, offering such a relationship is the kind of support most clearly linked to positive health outcomes.

Most patients judge respect, understanding and honesty to be very helpful. For example, in one study of cancer patients, over 90% of the participants mentioned this kind of moral support as being among the most helpful aid received from friends and family.

Assisting With Decision Making

- When my mother was hospitalized I helped her consider the "pros and cons of radiation therapy [and we spent time] planning for the future."
- After my friend was assaulted, we would talk about what happened and "how he was going to resolve the problem."

Decision-making support is closely related to the offer of a positive relationship. If the patient is capable of making rational judgments, you can best provide decision-making support by serving as a problem-solving consultant.

In the belief they are helping the person, friends and familiy members sometimes try to remove decision-making responsibility from a clearheaded patient. But such overprotectiveness has been shown to exacerbate symptoms. For instance, over-protective spouses have been shown to discourage full participation in the hospital regimen and thereby prolong recovery.

But while overprotectiveness has been shown to be unhealthy, recognizing autonomy and encouraging creative problem solving have been shown to foster positive patient outcomes. The next few paragraphs describe how you can encourage adaptive decision making on the part of the patient.

Think of problem solving as having three phases— exploring thoughts and feelings, considering alternatives, and developing a plan.

Exploring thoughts and feelings is the first step in being a problem-solving consultant. The objective is to clarify the patient's concerns using the kind of positive relationship discussed in the previous section. A shared feeling of understanding is your goal. You accomplish this by reflecting the major ideas and emotions communicated by the patient and by asking an occasional question. You have explored sufficiently when no new concerns emerge or when the patient begins to cover the same topics again. When either of these occur, you can wrap up this phase by summarizing the crucial concerns and feelings that have been shared.

Considering alternatives is the second step in problem solving. There are a couple of ways you can accomplish this phase. One is to use a brainstorming approach in which you encourage the patient to generate a large number of options without critically evaluating any of them. Simply have the person name a possibility and then go on to another one. After exhausting the patient's ready supply of ideas, go back and consider the two or three best-sounding possibilities.

Another approach is to focus on just a few options. You can begin by discussing what the person already has tried, then move to a consideration of what the patient has thought about, and, finally, ask the person what other options might be possible. Once you have encouraged this kind of input from the patient, it may be appropriate to mention an idea that you believe might work. But such a suggestion should be low-key and should come as a last resort.

As with brainstorming, the object of this approach is to consider in detail two or three possibilities. Once you have selected an idea to examine closely, have the person think about the advantages and disadvantages of the option. Be sure to include a critique of practical factors associated with implementing the idea.

Should the person come up with an option that you believe is unwise, you have the choice of being judgmental or nonjudgmental. If you choose to be judgmental you simply tell the person what you think of the idea. Unfortunately, the results from this approach may be temporary—the person may agree with you while you are there and then implement the bad idea once you are gone. Consequently, it often is more effective to be nonjudgmental and to encourage the patient to fully explore the likely results of the action. If it really is a bad idea, the person probably will reject it after fully realizing the negative consequences. But unlike the rejection of an idea in response to your criticism, this rejection is likely to last.

As with the exploration phase, once alternatives have been considered it should be possible for you to summarize what has been covered. You can name the two or three most prominent options and briefly cite the major pros and cons associated with each one.

Developing a plan is the final phase of problem solving. The objective is to select an option or a combination of options. Regardless of the alternatives selected, the plan will be a good one if it has four characteristics.

- [ ] It is *negotiated*. You contribute your common sense and your experience, but the plan's developement is a joint effort. You do not tell the person what to do.
- [ ] It is *specific*. The patient can describe the concrete actions necessary to implement the plan, and there are ways to verify that the strategy is working.
- [ ] It is *realistic*. It actually is possible for the patient to accomplish the tasks involved in the plan, and the goal is likely to be reached. The patient must have the strength and energy needed to carry out the plan.
- [ ] It is focused in the *present*. There are at least some initial steps that the person can do today or tomorrow to begin implementing the plan.

When I visit a friend or loved one in the hospital I keep in mind the importance of offering a positive relationship and decision-making support. For instance, last night I visited a friend in the hospital. My wife and I know her because we attend the same church. She has been a member for about two years, and most of our interactions have been in that setting. I would not characterize our relationship as either long-standing or especially close. But we do care about her and we want her to get better.

Although I had called in the afternoon and arranged to come after she expected to be finished with dinner, she still was eating when we arrived. Consequently, we offered to sit off to the side as she finished her meal. When she got to the dessert she asked us to join her, and we talked as she ate. After finishing her meal she offered to take us to the dayroom of the ward, and we followed as she led the way. Upon arriving, we sat at a card table and then had about a 20-minute discussion. We listened to what she had to say, reflected our understanding, and, from time to time, asked her to clarify a point she was trying to make. A few times we shared experiences from our own lives that seemed similar to the issues she was discussing. We helped her to evaluate possible consequences of actions she was considering, but we did not tell her what to do or criticize her decisions. By the end of the interaction she had developed a plan that she intended to implement the next morning.

During our visit she shared intimate details of her life that we never had known. She also expressed concerns about her medical care and home situation, then considered ways of handling those concerns. It was the most frank discussion we had ever had with her. At the end of the visit she sincerely thanked us for coming, and my wife and I both felt good about having seen her.

I believe her self-disclosure during our visit was due primarily to the support we offered. We demonstrated respect in two ways: by letting her decide when and where the visit should take place, and by discussing her past and future behavior without being critical. We conveyed understanding by reflecting the essential thoughts and feelings she communicated, and we showed her that that we could be trusted by being honest in our reactions, while also disclosing some information about ourselves.

The plan she developed came about as a result of our decision-making support. By getting her thoughts and feelings out in the open and by considering her options, she was able to develop a negotiated, specific, realistic and present-oriented plan.

Typical concerns were expressed by our friend. For instance, she questioned some of her doctor's decisions. Her criticism was consistent with my survey of hospital patients. When I asked patients to describe the most negative apect of their hospital stay, by far the most frequent response was dissatisfaction with the staff.

Wait! Don't jump to an incorrect conclusion. You should know that I also asked the patients to describe the most positive aspect of their stay. In response to that question, the most frequent answer was the care and concern provided by the staff. So just like family and friends, staff members are either part of the problem or part of the solution. You will find that Chapter 5 contains most of my comments concerning hospital staff.

The second most frequently mentioned problem in my survey was represented by comments like these.

- "I was bored."
- "It got pretty lonely at times."
- "...boredom."

Feelings of isolation and boredom are difficulties that family and friends can do a great deal to counteract. You will decrease these feelings by supporting the patient in any of the ways previously discussed.

The third most frequently cited concern was difficulties with other patients.

- The most negative aspect of my hospital stay was "an inconsiderate, noisy roommate. If I got a phone call while I was asleep or out of the room, I would never get the message."
- "My roommate didn't seem too sane. [He] went wild one night and tore all his tubes out and was walking around the room looking for some clothes so he could leave."
- "The room next to mine had very loud patients...television and visitors."

If your friend or relative is having difficulties with a roommate, other patient, or visitor, it may be appropriate to discuss the patient's concerns using the problem-solving format. It probably will be better for the person to develop a plan for coping with the situation, rather than continuing to fret about it.

Other problem areas that patients commonly mention include hospital food, the length of visits and the number of visitors. You also can assist the person in developing ways to deal with these kinds of concerns.

Some patients are not capable of making rational choices. The person may be unconscious, semiconscious or otherwise incapable of clearheaded thinking. Patient involvement in problem solving is not possible at those times. Instead, it will be necessary for others to make decisions for the person.

The medical staff has responsibility for many of the decisions that must be made. But it is also a good idea for a close friend or family member to be available for decision-making support.

It is best for the patient to select such an advocate during a period of clearheaded thinking. If the hospitalization has been planned, such a decision may be possible before admission. Even if the hospital stay was unplanned, there may be an opportunity after admission for the patient to select an advocate.

In cases where the patient has not chosen an advocate, others may need to make that decision for the person. In the absence of patient input, selecting an advocate may be more difficult. But the inability of the patient to make the choice means that the selection of an advocate is crucial. Friends, family members and the hospital staff all may participate in choosing a person to represent the patient's interests.

The patient's needs are the top priority for the advocate. If the patient wants a point of view represented to the staff, and is unable to communicate the message, it is the responsibility of the advocate to transmit that viewpoint for the person.

It also is the responsibility of the advocate to use common sense. If something seems unreasonable or ill-advised, then the advocate should think twice before acting on the request. Such a decision is easier to make if there is one primary advocate who has kept up with the course of the patient's hospitalization. Judging what is reasonable is much more difficult when an individual has had only spotty contact with events.

If there is surgery, the advocate should plan to be at the hospital during the operation and recovery period. The medical team should know who the advocate is and where the person can be found in the hospital. Knowing the advocate's identity and location will enable the staff to contact the person, if that becomes necessary.

Should the patient be taken to a special care unit, it will not be possible for the advocate to be available all of the time. But the friend or family member should learn how to contact the unit for status reports. For instance, calling the patient's primary nurse often is a good strategy.

Conversely, the special unit staff should be able to contact the advocate. The person's location and phone number (if applicable) can be left with the unit staff.

When the plan calls for the patient to return to a regular hospital room, the advocate should plan to be there when the patient arrives. It is necessary for the advocate to know when the patient is expected back in the room. In the minority of cases where the patient does not return within the expected time frame, the advocate should investigate the reason for the delay. The first place to check is the nurses' station; it is appropriate for a nurse or a clerk to call and find out patient's location and status. In the rare case when such calls fail to generate sufficient information, the next person to contact is the patient's attending physician.

When the patient does return to the room, it is best if the advocate can stay until the patient is clearheaded. Being available during this period makes it easier for the patient to transmit wishes to the staff. For instance, one patient said "The most important visitor was my friend who stayed all day immediately after the operation. She didn't talk but was able to give me what I needed, call the nurse, etc."

You now have read about five kinds of support, roughly in order from least to most difficult. Any friend or family member can provide information and can give appropriate gifts. It is fairly easy to offer news of interest and to bring an appreciated present.

There are certain tasks with which most visitors can help, while other duties require some degree of intimacy before a patient will feel comfortable accepting assistance. Be willing to lend a hand if it is appropriate.

Moral support comes in a variety of forms, no doubt some more suitable for you than others. You must judge whether you should talk about pleasant times, joke with the patient, or offer prayer and scripture. But I strongly recommend that you do strive to convey honesty, respect and understanding.

Should these three skills characterize your interaction, you will be in a position to serve as a problem-solving consultant. With a clearheaded patient you can explore concerns, consider options and develop plans. If the person is unable to think clearly, you or someone else may need to serve as an advocate for the patient's interests.

Your effectiveness as a visitor often depends upon what you say. The next chapter takes a look at the pros and cons associated with the six most frequently used helping responses.

3
Choosing Your Response

Certain ways of wording thoughts are better than others. This chapter describes communication techniques that can help you effectively offer moral and decision-making support.

You may want to skip the chapter for now if responding to uncertainty or helping with problem solving will not be part of your next visit. You also may wish to go on the Chapter 4 if you already possess good communication skills.

If you have decided to read Chapter 3, get ready to reevaluate the way you normally say things. It will be helpful to start by identifying your current opinions about several ways of responding to a patient. All of the approaches to be discussed are represented in the following exercise. It begins with an exchange between you and a patient, then lists ten possible ways you could respond. For each of the ten options, put a mark somewhere on the hindering/helpful line.

Here is the beginning dialogue.

You: How are things going?
Patient: OK right now. But I'm really feeling uneasy about having a general anesthetic tomorrow; I know some people are put to sleep and don't wake up. Maybe I really don't need this operation.

Choosing Your Response

What might you say next? For each of the ten possibilities listed, put a vertical mark somewhere on the hindering/helpful line.

A. What might happen if you didn't have the operation?

hindering _____ helpful

B. Are you scheduled for surgery in the morning?

hindering _____ helpful

C. It's scary to think about what might happen tomorrow.

hindering _____ helpful

D. I'm sorry you're worried.

hindering _____ helpful

E. You probably feel this way because the anesthesiologist hasn't been by to talk with you.

hindering _____ helpful

F. You should try to think about something besides the operation.

hindering _____ helpful

G. I'm sure everything will be all right.

hindering _____ helpful

H. How could you ease your mind? What does your doctor say about the risk?

hindering _____ helpful

I. You aren't really thinking of backing out, are you?

hindering _____ helpful

J. Why haven't you told anyone you felt this way?

hindering _____ helpful

Having considered ten possible responses, here are some patient opinions about the response styles of their visitors.

- The most negative aspect of having visitors was "repeating all of the details of the tests, etc. each time someone new came. It was very tiring."
- The worst part of seeing visitors was "having them ask questions all the time. It gets boring after awhile."
- Visitors "asked me questions [when] I couldn't talk. [They should] ask very few questions."
- The worst part of having visitors was "having to repeat my condition over and over....[I didn't like answering questions about] the details of my health down to what I had to eat."
- "It can be tedious as well as depressing to repeat the story of my condition for the hundredth time."
- I didn't like "having them ask questions all the time. It was tiring after awhile."
- Friends and family should "respect feelings about my being there and try to understand."
- Visitors "should show more empathy towards [patients]."
- "It is important to hear what patients have on their minds and give them a chance to release negative feelings."
- The most positive aspect of having visitors was "being able to verbalize my feelings about the surgery."
- "They kept saying I was going home and I'd still be there the next day."
- The most negative aspect of visits was "having visitors feel sorry for me."
- I didn't like "expressions of pity or sympathy."
- "I hope they won't pity me."
- Visitors "should not try to play doctor and tell you what they would do if they were you."

- Visitors "shouldn't lie to me by telling me things about my health that aren't true."
- "Sometimes you would just rather...not try to keep talking about why you're in."

You now have read several patient opinions, and you have thought about ten specific replies that one might make to a patient. The ten options in the opening exercise represent six modes of response. Five of the choices are examples of interrogation, and there is one example each of reflection, sympathy, analysis, advice and reassurance. By examining each of the options in the exercise, the remainder of the chapter considers pros and cons associated with these six common ways of responding to patients.

Interrogation

Response A "What might happen if you didn't have the operation?"

Open-ended questions such as response A begin with the words "what" or "how." They identify broad areas to be discussed. Such questions allow the person a considerable amount of freedom in deciding upon the exact nature and amount of information to be revealed. While specifying a topic, they allow the patient to choose material that seems the most relevant. Open-ended questions are appropriate if the individual possesses the information in which you are interested and feels comfortable discussing it with you.

If you want to respond with a question in the opening exercise, then option A is a good form of interrogation. It identifies an area to be discussed, while still giving the patient a good deal of freedom in expressing thoughts and feelings.

After being admitted to a patient's room and introducing yourself, one way to begin the interaction is with a sincere "How are you doing today?" or "How are things going?" I especially like the second question, because it gives the person a great deal of freedom in responding. The patient can answer by talking about current feelings or by giving a less revealing response. If in reply you get a standard "fine" or "OK," you may want to narrow the focus a bit. For instance, you might say "How are the tests going?" or "What will be happening today?"

Response B "Are you scheduled for surgery in the morning?"

Closed questions, such as response B, are useful when you want to be more specific than a "what" or "how" question will allow. For example, you might want to know whether the attending physician has seen the patient today. If you know the physician usually visits patients between 7:00 a.m. and 9:00 a.m., you might ask "How did things go this morning?" In describing the morning, the patient might include an account of the doctor's visit. But if the information in which you are interested is not contained in the patient's reply to your open-ended question, you can acknowledge the person's answer then follow with a closed question.

Closed questions specify a precise area of information and the patient's response usually can be a simple "yes" or "no." For example, "Did Dr. Johnson stop by to see you this morning?" As this question demonstrates, closed questions commonly begin with "is," "did," "have" or "does." Closed questions serve a purpose; they allow you to request a very small bit of information. But their advantage also can be a disadvantage. Since only a small amount of specific information may be provided, closed questions are not an efficient means of generating discussion. If they are used frequently the patient is likely to fall into a pattern of brief, limited responses. The person will wait for the next question rather than try to initiate discussion of a topic.

In the opening exercise, I believe response B is inappropriate. As presented in the dialogue, the patient expresses a willingness to discuss certain matters. A closed question as the next response may result in less sharing by the person. I believe finding out whether tomorrow's surgery will be in the morning is not worth risking a decrease in patient input. In this example, it is more important to encourage the patient to continue discussing concerns. When a person is opening up in this way, it usually is best to avoid closed questions. There probably will be a time later in the visit when you can ask for needed information.

Sequences of questions can allow the effective use of both open and closed questions. It is best to begin with an open-ended question if the patient has the information you want and is interested in discussing it with you. When you need a more specific response you then can ask a closed question. This is called a *funnel sequence* because you begin with wide-open questions and progressively narrow your focus. The following is an example of a funnel sequence.

"How have things been going since you were admitted?"
"What happened this morning?"
"Did you have some difficulty with the procedure?"

But what if the person is reluctant to talk with you or needs guidance in discussing the desired topic? In either of these instances, the *inverted funnel* sequence of questions can be very helpful. This approach is the opposite of the funnnel sequence; rather than beginning with a broad question, you start by requesting a small bit of information. Giving the patient some direction by asking specific questions may help the person feel more at ease and more willing to open up as the interaction progresses. When the patient's answers become more expansive you can widen the focus of your questions. Here is an example of the inverted funnel sequence.

"Did you go for therapy this morning?"
"What did the therapist say about your progress?"
"How are you feeling about the therapy?"

There are advantages and disadvantages to asking questions. I believe that at times it is appropriate to ask for information, and the preceding paragraphs describe some helpful ways to use questions. But remember that the heading for this section is **Interrogation.**

What comes to mind when you think of the word "interrogation"?

An image that occurs to me is from an old gangster movie. Two police detectives are in an interrogation room with a prisoner. There is a small table with a shaded light bulb hanging over it. The prisoner is seated at the table and one of the detectives is standing next to it. While the prisoner's face is illuminated by the glare of the light, only the detective's midsection can be seen clearly; his shoulders and head are merely an outline in the shadows. The other detective is not seen at all, but you know he is there because he occasionally fires a question.

I believe it is useful to keep such an image in mind whenever you ask questions. Asking for information has its place, but you do not want to come across as an interrogator who follows one question with another.

Reflection

Response C "It's scary to think about what might happen tomorrow."

Acknowledging the patient's comments is essential to a helpful visit. Some of your acknowledgment can be nonverbal expressions of interest such as making frequent eye contact and occasionally saying "mmhmm" or "unhuh." But you also should demonstrate your understanding through reflection.

This technique involves summarizing the essential thoughts and feelings just communicated by the patient and rephrasing them in your own words. It demonstrates your understanding of the person, and, as discussed in the last chapter, communicating such understanding is an essential aspect of a positive relationship. The empathy you show through reflection is a tangible demonstration of interest and caring that can contribute to a patient's sense of belonging.

Reflection is an excellent way to keep the interaction focused on topics the patient wants to discuss. For instance, sometimes a patient may wish to talk about concerns and feelings regarding medical issues, while at other times the person may want to avoid such topics. Reflection allows you to be responsive to the patient's wishes. It conveys an attitude of receptiveness and attention, while most of the interchange continues to originate from the other person.

For example, you say "How are things going?" and the person says "Today is the day the test results are supposed to be back. I want to know what they are, but I'm afraid to find out. I just hope they aren't too bad." You respond by saying "Waiting to hear is really hard." In this case, the patient wants to discuss medically related feelings and concerns, and you follow the person's lead by using a reflective response.

At another time you might ask "How are things going?" and

the patient might say "I'm so glad you're here. Do you remember last Memorial Day? I was just thinking about that trip we took. We got some great pictures. Every time I look at those photos I start thinking of the good times we had that day." You respond by saying "It's fun to think about that day again." In this instance, the patient wants to avoid current medical concerns and you respect the person's wishes by using an appropriate reflective response.

Let's say you ask how things are going and you don't understand the patient's reply. Maybe you need the patient to repeat part of the response or perhaps you want a medical term explained. In any case, if you do not understand the person it is appropriate to ask for clarification. Be willing to seek more information rather than pretending you understand when you really don't.

Remember that offering a positive relationship requires that you be honest in what you say. Feigned comprehension does not help the patient and may set the stage for an embarrassing situation later on, should your lack of understanding be discovered inadvertently.

When you make a reflective statement such as "It sounds like the procedure was more painful than you expected," you are communicating what you believe the patient to be saying and you are giving the person an opportunity to modify your perception, should the patient wish to do so. Let's imagine the person responds by saying "No, it really didn't hurt; it was more like a feeling of strong pressure." Even if you miss the mark like this once in a while, you still can be fostering good communication. When a patient disagrees with your reflection the person probably will point out the discrepancy. This usually allows you to get a better idea of the individual's true feelings. So reflection can enhance understanding even when you make a mistake.

Sometimes you may accurately reflect a patient's concern but the person may claim not to be worried about that issue. This is an example of denial. Such self-deception probably should not be challenged if there is nothing the patient could do about the concern anyway. There is no sense in confronting the person's denial if a successful challenge will only distress the patient without leading to any change in the circumstances. On the other hand, it may be appropriate to reiterate your perception of the patient's situation if the denial is preventing the person from taking action in areas where adaptive change is possible.

Reflection is a valuable response whenever there is a need to change attitudes and behavior. Remember that exploring thoughts and feelings is the first step in problem solving. By conveying understanding and acceptance, you are helping the person to explore and to organize ideas and emotions. Having accurately assessed the situation the individual is in a better position to decide upon a course of action.

Reflection can occur at several emotional levels.

☐ You can summarize the factual information communicated by the patient. This kind of reflection conveys a superficial level of understanding and encourages the person to continue surveying the situation.

☐ In addition to information, you also may reflect feelings described by the individual. Reflection of emotions usually results in the patient feeling more fully understood and more willing to discuss the situation in greater detail.

☐ If you reflect feelings that are not expressly stated by the person, you move to a deeper level of understanding; exploration becomes more detailed and intense. At this level, the patient may not be aware of the emotions being communicated until you reflect the behavior that signals their existence.

Here is an example of how the same statement could be reflected at three different levels. "After spending two weeks in the hospital, I won't be in good enough shape to see my daughter in the tennis tournament. I'm really going to miss that, and I know she was counting on me." At an information level a reflective response could be, "Your physical condition will keep you from going." At a surface feeling level a response could be, "It's frustrating to be out of commission." A reflection of underlying feelings could be, "You blame yourself for letting her down."

In general, effective communication can be achieved best by matching or slightly exceeding the depth of feeling conveyed by the person. The information level ignores the feeling component, while the underlying feeling level is really just an educated guess about what is on the person's mind. Sticking to surface feeling reflections probably is the most conducive to effective communication with the patient.

When you first try reflection you may feel that you are "doing nothing"; but, it is "doing something" for two reasons. First, it is helpful, as can be seen in the other person's behavior. The individual frequently expands upon the message reflected by further discussing thoughts and feelings. Second, reflection takes effort on your part. You must hear, understand, remember, summarize, and rephrase the message received. Perfectly performing each of these functions and being on target all of the time is impossible. But remember that reflection allows you to be human and make mistakes. When you misunderstand the person, it will be obvious because you will incorrectly reflect the message being communicated—thereby giving the patient an opportunity to correct your perceptions and to clarify the issue.

There is one situation in which your reflection should be limited. If the patient is depressed it is appropriate to acknowledge the sadness with a couple of reflections, but you do not want to continue reflecting the person's low mood. Multiple reflections centering on hopelessness or helplessness will create a downward spiral of depression. As the interaction progresses, both you and the patient will feel worse if you continue to reflect the person's despondency.

It is better to use a couple of reflections that show you understand the patient is feeling down, then go on to a discussion of what can be done about the person's situation. The problem-solving approach discussed in the last chapter is an appropriate response to a patient who is depressed.

When your intent is to encourage communication from the patient, it usually is most productive to use a mixture of reflection, open-ended questions and closed questions. Even if the patient is reluctant to express concerns, the right combination of these responses can encourage the person to share thoughts and feelings with you.

In my own experience, suicidal teenagers often are reluctant to talk. But reflection and appropriate questions have served me well in encouraging these young people to tell me what is on their minds. In one case, a 16-year-old girl was hospitalized after attempting suicide by taking an overdose of medication. The day after she was admitted, her physician asked me to visit her. The following is an an account of how that interaction began.

Visitor: "Knock, knock."
Patient: No response.
Visitor: (The door is open and the patient is laying on the bed staring at the ceiling. I walk over to the bed.) "I'm Dr. France. I'm a psychologist. Dr. Matthews asked me to stop by and see you. How are you doing this morning?"
Patient: She responds by turning away from me.

Visitor: (My open-ended question having failed, I resort to an inverted funnel sequence.) "Did Dr. Matthews see you this morning?"
Patient: "Yeah."
Visitor: "Did he say when he thought you would be going home?" (closed question)
Patient: "Yeah."
Visitor: "When did he say you would be leaving the hospital?" (closed question)
Patient: "Tomorrow."
Visitor: "So you will just be here one more day." (information level reflection)
Patient: "Yeah."
Visitor: "What do you think about being here?" (open-ended question)
Patient: "I don't know."
Visitor: (My "what" question had not elicited much of a response so I decided to go back to a closed question.) "Did you eat something this morning?"
Patient: "Yeah."
Visitor: "What did you have?" (fairly specific open-ended question)
Patient: "An egg and some bread."
Visitor: "How was it?" (open-ended question)
Patient: "It was awful. The egg was all runny and cold."
Visitor: "So, you didn't like breakfast very much." (surface feeling reflection)
Patient: "Yeah, it was about as bad as that stuff they gave me last night to make me throw up."
Visitor: "I guess being forced to vomit like that was unpleasant. How are you feeling this morning?" (a reflection followed by an open-ended question—often a good combination to use)
Patient: "I feel tired and my stomach is sore. I just want to go home."
Visitor: "You've been through the wringer and you are ready to leave." (surface feeling reflection)
Patient: "Yeah. I just want to get out of here. I'm OK. They got out of me everything I swallowed. I don't understand why they say I have

to stay until tomorrow. If I'm OK now they should let me go."
Visitor: "So you're all right and ready to go home." (surface feeling reflection)
Patient: "Yeah. But I guess home won't be much better. They're always telling me what to do—just like the people here have been ordering me around."
Visitor: "You don't like it when people tell you what to do." (surface feeling reflection)
Patient: "That's right. That's how I ended up here in the first place...."

Most hospitalized patients are not nearly so reluctant to talk as was this person. I described my interaction with her in order to demonstrate how you can use reflection and appropriate questions to encourage even a reticent patient to open up with you. By relying upon these techniques you can explore the nature of the individual's concerns. In so doing, you will be demonstrating interest and empathy. Demonstrating to the patient that you care and want to understand can help the person cope with the hospital experience.

Here is another example of a visitor-patient interaction.

Visitor: "How are things going today?"
Patient: "Fine."
Visitor: "How is your leg doing after the surgery?"
Patient: "Well, it's pretty sore, but the doctor says that is normal. I guess I expected my leg to hurt some, but I didn't think I would be having trouble with my hand."
Visitor: "Your hand is bothering you."
Patient: "Kind of. You know when your hand goes to sleep and you feel all those little pin prickles. Well that is the way my left hand feels all the time. I move it around but that feeling doesn't go away."
Visitor: "Well, I'm sorry to hear that. I had the same thing when I had my surgery. They probably injured your elbow when you were asleep during the operation. There really is not much that can be done

about it, but you should tell your doctor. It will take a few months, but my problem went away and I'm sure yours will too."

This visitor started out using two open-ended questions and a reflection. The patient eventually responded by sharing the concern about his hand. But once hearing that concern, the visitor jumped in with a reply that included four common kinds of responses: sympathy, analysis, advice and reassurance. All of these responses can have detrimental effects on the interaction, so let's take a closer look at them.

Sympathy

Response D "I'm sorry you're worried."

You are describing how you feel when you make a statement like "I'm sorry you're worried" or "I'm sorry to hear that." Such expressions of sympathy probably constitute the most frequent response to individuals who are in distress.

If your intent is to talk about how you are feeling—rather than how the patient is feeling—and you pity the person, then it may be appropriate to express sympathy. Although a sympathetic statement such as response D can communicate pity to the patient, it does not do much else. And, like the patient quoted at the beginning of the chapter, being pitied is something few patients want. Pity places the patient in an inferior status and can contribute to feelings of decreased autonomy and dignity. If these are not outcomes you desire, you should avoid sympathy in favor of other responses previously discussed.

Analysis

Response E "You probably feel this way because the anesthesiologist hasn't been by to talk with you."

Describing the underlying cause of an occurrence is the intent of analytical statements such as response E and "They probably injured your elbow when you were asleep during the operation." Analysis is intended to explain how events developed and what they mean. As with sympathy, analysis changes the focus of the interaction from what the patient has to share to what the visitor has to say.

I believe response E is inappropriate for a number of reasons.

- ☐ It is a guess. There is no evidence in the dialogue that the anesthesiologist has not talked with the patient.
- ☐ The response is condescending. It implies the patient is stupid for being afraid.
- ☐ The timing is wrong. The patient obviously wants to talk, but response E shifts the interaction away from what that person has to say.

Nevertheless, I believe there are times when analysis can be helpful. For example, the following dialogue demonstrates how I believe analysis can be appropriate and useful.

Patient: "The pain is not so bad as long as I am talking with someone or listening to one of the comedy tapes you brought me. But when I try to go to sleep the pain gets worse. It doesn't make any sense to me and it really makes it hard to get some sleep."
Visitor: "These fluctuations in the pain seem mysterious to you, and they are making it difficult for you to sleep." (surface feeling reflection)
Patient: "That's right."

(What the patient described—and the visitor acknowledged through reflection—is a kind of pain that subsides when the person focuses attention on other things and gets worse when there is not distracting stimulation. It is caused by sensory nerve stimulation and it is discussed in the next chapter. A visitor who knows about sensory nerve pain could make the following comment.)

Visitor: "I've read about pain like that. If your sensory nerves are signaling pain but your mind is occupied with something else, your brain ignores a lot of those pain signals. But during quiet times, like when you try to fall asleep, your brain has less activity so it pays more attention to the painful stimulation, and the pain gets worse." (analysis)
Patient: "Well, that's interesting, but what do I do to get some sleep?"
Visitor: "What has your doctor told you to do when the pain starts to get worse?" (open-ended question that puts responsibility back on the patient)

This analysis let's the patient know that the pain makes sense, given the person's particular circumstances. Notice though that analysis does not magically solve the problem, but it can lead to a consideration of what to do about the difficulty. Understanding how things got to be the way they are may encourage the person to do something about the situation. In the example above, taking the mystery out of the pain fluctuations leads the patient to focus on "What do I do to get some sleep?" Having achieved some insight into the causes of the pain fluctuations, the person is ready to decide upon a course of action.

Even if you choose to analyze the patient's condition, you should return the focus to the person's thoughts and feelings as soon as possible. You want to continue doing all you can to foster the patient's autonomy and control.

Whenever you use analysis you are making a judgment, which can be risky—especially if you are basing your conclusion on incomplete information. For example, I recently visited a friend who had a malignant kidney tumor necessitating removal of the kidney. During a presurgery test, she suffered cardiac arrest but was revived. Because of that episode there was a question as to whether she could withstand the process of having the kidney removed. The decision regarding surgery would be made the next day. While I was in the room, she had the following conversation with another visitor.

Visitor: "How long will you be here?"
Patient: "I don't know. I might go home tomorrow."
Visitor: "If they're letting you go home you must be doing OK."
Patient: "I don't think they've decided how I'm doing."
Visitor: "Well I think it's terrific that you may be going home."

For my friend, going home would be a bad sign—not a good one. The visitor's analysis of the situation was inaccurate and merely demonstrated that she did not fully understand the circumstances.

Advice

Response F "You should try to think about something besides the operation."

You are deciding on a course of action for the patient when you make a statement such as response F or "You should tell your doctor." Patients usually believe that advice from their doctors is helpful, but, as mentioned in the last chapter, patients generally do not like medical advice when it comes from family members or friends.

The intent of giving advice is to tell the other person what to do, but advice may have more far-reaching effects than merely providing a course of action. If you make a statement such as "You should take your pain medication," you are saying that you are in a better position than the patient to decide what should be done. Feeling overprotected in this way robs one's autonomy and can lead to feelings of humiliation and resentment. When you establish yourself as the decision maker, you also move the focus of the exchange to your ideas and decrease the person's willingness to freely discuss topics.

Advice can turn out to be a "no win" situation. For instance, let's say the patient believes the suggestion is inappropriate; not only is the person likely to reject it, but the individual also may conclude that you do not understand the circumstances. On the other hand, what if your advice is accepted but then fails to produce the desired results? In that case the patient may blame you for the lack of success. The most positive outcome possible is for the advice to be accepted and to be used successfully. But even that outcome can lead to difficulties, since the next time a problem arises the patient may sit back and wait for you to solve it.

In my opinion response F is inappropriate on several counts.

☐ The dialogue does not suggest advice is necessary. There is no evidence that the patient is incapable of generating options.
☐ The advice given is easy to say but hard to implement. It fails to recognize the difficulties of the situation.
☐ The timing is wrong. As with response D and E, it is much too early to change the focus away from what this patient has to share.

Choosing Your Response

Recognizing that advice can have a variety of dangers associated with it, there are times when it may be appropriate to offer a suggestion. Giving advice is acceptable if the patient is unable to think of a solution or if the plan the person comes up with does not seem to be a good idea. In either of those instances, it may be helpful for you to throw out a possibility that you believe would have a good chance of working. But remember, when you offer advice you risk a variety of undesirable outcomes, including having your idea rejected, being accused of not understanding, being blamed if the plan fails, and fostering dependency.

The following dialogue presents a situation in which it might be appropriate to give advice.

Patient: "I don't see why my doctor won't let me get out of bed to use the bathroom. I hate trying to use this bedpan. Things would be a lot easier if I could just walk over to the bathroom."
Visitor: "You're really annoyed about being restricted to your bed." (surface feeling reflection)
Patient: "Yeah. In fact, I'm not going to put up with it. I can walk to the bathroom. So that's what I'm going to do."
Visitor: "You are so fed up that you want to ignore your doctor's orders." (surface feeling reflection)
Patient: "That's right. I'm going to do it. They can't keep me in bed."
Visitor: "Well, walking to the bathroom on your own is one possibility. But I'm a little worried about you. What would you think about asking one of the nurses if she could arrange for you to get to the bathroom?" (information level reflection, self-disclosure, followed by advice)

This advice risks all of the dangers mentioned above. But getting the patient to consider asking the nurse for help may be preferable to the person going ahead with the original plan.

Reassurance

Response G "I'm sure everything will be all right."

Decreasing distress is the intent of statements such as response G and "My problem went away and I'm sure yours will too." These are examples of reassurance. The goal of such comments is to reduce the patient's concern with assurances that things are not that bad. But reassurance implies you do not understand the situation if you base your comment on how you would like things to be rather than on the facts of the case. Patients are not fooled by statements like response G; instead, they see them as unhelpful. Offering false hope merely suggests that you want to avoid the real issues.

If you really do have information that supports a good prognosis, then reassurance may be appropriate. The following dialogue offers an example of such an instance.

Patient: "They took me to surgery for my arm. That must mean my elbow is in pretty bad shape. I wonder if I am going to have permanent damage?"
Visitor: "You're unsure about how things are looking for your elbow, and that's troubling. Have you seen the surgeon since your operation?" (surface feeling reflection followed by a closed question)
Patient: "They tell me he came by but that I was asleep."
Visitor: "Well, I talked with him a little after the operation. He said it was too early to say for sure, but that things went well during the surgery and that the X rays looked good."

Such a fact-based reassurance is not likely to work miracles, but it is appropriate and may help put the patient's mind at ease. Just be sure to avoid embellishing such assurances with how you would like things to be.

When Communication Is Difficult

Sometimes the patient's condition makes talking difficult. When this is the case, writing may be a possibility. In such instances, making a note pad available might be the best aid to communication. (See the Intensive Care Unit section of Chapter 6 for further discussion of communication aids.)

Whatever the person's condition, a note pad can enhance privacy. If there are other patients in the room, a note pad allows you to communicate in confidence with the person you are visiting.

If the patient's medical condition makes it difficult to talk, relying on closed questions is another good technique for gaining information. The person will be better able to respond to queries that can be answered "yes" or "no," or that require some other minimal response. For example, "Were you able to keep your breakfast down?" "Did you see Dr. Martin this morning?" or "When did you have your last pain medicine?"

There are several kinds of questions you should avoid, especially when it is difficult for the patient to respond. These are multiple questions, leading questions and "why" questions.

Response H "How could you ease your mind? What does your doctor say about the risk?"

Multiple questions are demonstrated in response H. They involve asking two or more things before giving the person a chance to respond. Rather than seeking clarification of what you mean, a patient finding it difficult to talk may answer just one of the questions you asked. If that occurs, you may not know which question is being answered. Multiple questions never are appropriate, but they can be especially annoying when it is difficult for the other person to respond. Other examples of multiple questions would be, "Did you tell the nurse about the problem or did you forget?" or "Are you feeling any better today? Did the pain medicine seem to help any? Do you want anything to drink?"

Response I "You aren't really thinking of backing out, are you?"

Leading questions, such as response I, seek agreement rather than a genuine reply from the person. They are biased; it is easier to give one answer than another. Like multiple questions, they always should be avoided, but their use can be especially detrimental to good communication when it is difficult for the other person to respond. Another example of a leading question would be, "You didn't like your lunch, did you?" Whether or not the patient liked the lunch, the easiest response is a negative one if talking is difficult.

Response J "Why haven't you told anyone you felt this way?"

"Why" questions require the person to analyze the situation. Often such questions are perceived as accusations or as scolding. A patient threatened by a "why" question may respond with a rationalization or may fabricate an answer in order not to appear stupid. Such distortions become all the more likely if the person doesn't have the energy to provide a full explanation. For example, "Why didn't you tell me you were coming into the hospital?" is not likely to generate a helpful response. Maybe the individual forgot to tell you or maybe the hospitalization was unexpected. But you probably will not find out the real reason if you put the person on the defensive with a "why" question.

If you believe you must know why something has happened, try asking "What was the reason for...?" Such a request for an explanation does not sound as accusatory as a "why" question and tends to generate a less defensive response.

What did you think of the chapter? Here are the comments of a nurse who read it: "I thought this chapter was especially helpful,...[but] this information could be overwhelming to someone who has never learned it before."

Having taught communication skills to lay persons and professionals, I agree with this nurse's comments. These are effective techniques, but many of them probably are new to you.

I encourage you to give them a try and see how the other person responds. You might start with reflection, since it is such a forgiving response when you do make a mistake.

Remember that even if you miss the mark with a reflective statement, you still can be fostering good communication. The most likely response to an incorrect reflection is for the other person to clarify the message. Consequently, even mistakes can contribute to the development of shared understanding.

As you become more adept with these techniques, they will merge with your own communication style. Eventually, you may not even notice you are using them.

Having examined support possibilities and response options, the next chapter discusses several specific considerations that are likely to enhance your hospital visit.

4

Hospital Visit Etiquette

Most patients have strong opinions about the do's and don'ts of hospital visits.

- The worst part of my hospital stay was "the visitors who insisted on coming in my room when I was so very sick."
- "Sometimes I was too sick to feel up to seeing anyone."
- "I do not want [visitors] to smoke around me."
- "It's difficult to visit when too many come at once. It's confusing and tiring."
- "Too many [visitors] came all at once. It was draining emotionally to have so much stimulation concentrated into 30 minutes and then everyone would be gone and that left an empty feeling to be suddenly left alone....I think hospital visitation can be overpowering for any patient and most visitors don't realize that they haven't been the only one to visit the patient. Two, four, six, etc. visitors begin to really add up and take its toll on the patient and can drain the patient physically and emotionally.I have been in the hospital when I resented visitors very much. I wanted time for only my immediate family and also for just my own feelings....I have also been hospitalized when I looked forward to friends and their...visits. So, I do not feel it is a good idea to visit a patient unless you are certain that visitors are welcomed."

Hospital Visit Etiquette

As you can see from these comments, well-intentioned hospital visits can have negative effects on patients. Fortunately, most of these difficulties can be avoided by planning before the visit, demonstrating respect during the visit, and staying an appropriate length of time.

Planning Before the Visit

- Sometimes visitors "came at the wrong time."
- The most negative aspect of seeing visitors was "not having much control of their coming and going."
- Visitors "never left me alone!"
- "I couldn't control when they'd come and very often I'd not be ready. There was no privacy. I had no place to call my own. I couldn't even cry in peace."
- "I know the first two days I didn't want to see anyone because I felt really bad. After the second day [following surgery] it was OK as long as they didn't stay long."
- "I didn't really want visitors to come some days because I was tired and I just wanted to be by myself."
- "After sedation I felt that I wanted to be alone."
- "I would prefer that only close family members visit when I am coming out of surgery or when I am very sick."
- "About 75% of my hospital stay I was so sick I didn't want to be bothered talking to anyone so I really only wanted to talk to my husband and children. It was an effort to be civil if alone with [other] visitors."

Choosing the right time to visit depends upon the patient's condition as well as your relationship with the person. For instance, following surgery a patient's top priorities usually are pain relief and rest. If your presence fosters those goals then you should be there—as in the case of one who patient told me, "My mother helped me get sleep which I really needed and had a hard time getting."

A postsurgery visit by a companion or close family member can provide valuable support. But if you do not fall into one of those categories it may be best to postpone your visit until the person is stronger.

In deciding whether now is a good time to visit, you should consider the following four questions. If you answer "yes" to any of them you ought to think twice before visiting the patient.

Will your visit embarrass the patient?

- "I did not want anyone near me when I was so sick—the first day or two after surgery. It bothered me a lot for people other than my family to come into the room and see me so sick."
- "I hated having to sit around in my p.j.'s and entertain visitors."
- The most negative aspect of seeing visitors was "having them come at embarrassing times, [for example, when I was] sitting on the portable toilet."
- The worst part of having visitors was "that I would tire out so easily and didn't want to show it."
- "He sat on my bed. I was embarrassed for him to see me in my gown and so sick."

Is the patient too weak to benefit from your visit?

- "After surgery simple things like talking will tire you and you will fall asleep on guests."
- "I was just too sick and weak to be participating in conversation."
- "I was not able to say much at first because I had just come out of the O.R."
- "Sometimes you're tired, especially after the operation, and you feel that you have to entertain [visitors]. There were times when I couldn't wait for visiting hours to be over."

- The most negative aspect of visits was "having someone come to visit when you wanted to rest."
- "I sometimes didn't feel well enough to talk."
- "I was usually too medicated to hold intelligent conversations for long periods of time."
- "Trying to talk with tubes in your throat" is very unpleasant.
- The most negative aspect of my hospital stay was "having to smile at visitors when I didn't feel like it."
- "Sometimes I was too tired to be a 'good hostess.'"

Will your visit keep the patient from needed sleep?

- "During the first two days I only wanted to sleep. It was difficult to remain awake long enough to talk."
- "I just wanted to sleep or be left alone."
- "Much of the time they were there I would have preferred to sleep."
- "Sometimes I felt like sleeping while [visitors] were there."
- "You really do not want someone trying to talk when you're trying to sleep."
- "I just wanted to sleep and rest."
- Visitors "took up time when sleep was needed."
- "Sometimes [visitors] won't let you go to sleep if you're not well."
- "They got there right after I was given sedatives and I wanted to sleep."
- "There were times when I wanted to sleep but visitors were there."
- "Sometimes I was sleeping and [visitors] woke me up."

If the patient is in pain, will your visit make matters worse?

- The most negative aspect of having visitors was that they "saw me when I was in pain, crying."
- "I had a severe headache which was a normal reaction from the test. I called my parents to tell them not to visit because I was really ill. That was the only day I did not want visitors."

- "Right after the operation I was always in pain and tired and often found it difficult to entertain."
- The best aspect of having visitors was that they "made me forget the pain I was having."
- I liked having visitors because they provided "distraction from discomfort."
- Family and friends "helped to get my mind off my pain."
- "Visitors...distracted [me] from thinking about my physical pain."

Pain is one area in which patients report sharply divided opinions about the helpfulness of visitors. So let's take a closer look at pain.

Sensory nerves signal the existence of pain in response to surgery, traumatic injury or tissue damaging disease. There are three common interventions that may reduce the resulting discomfort.

☐ **Medication** often is appropriate with sensory pain. When used properly, pain reducing drugs can be both safe and effective.

☐ **Distraction** can help, as demonstrated by the last four patient comments. For a receptive patient, your visit may take the person's mind off the pain and thereby activate physiological mechanisms that can reduce discomfort.

You probably have experienced the pain reducing effects of distraction. Think of a time when you suffered an injury during a physically demanding task but you continued the activity. (Examples include athletic competition and manual labor.) Recall how much the injury hurt during the activity as compared to how it felt after you finished. You probably remember that the pain got worse when you completed the endeavor. The most common reason for such an increase in discomfort is that your mind no longer is distracted by the task, thereby worsening the pain.

Pain signaled from sensory nerves tends to cause greater discomfort during quiet times, such as when the patient tries to fall asleep. Consequently, the person may need an increase in pain medication when there is a decrease in distraction.

☐ **Information** can decrease anxiety and lessen pain. Providing ample information about an impending stressful experience can reduce discomfort during the procedure itself. The key word here is *ample*. Too little information may raise questions that are not sufficiently answered, with the result being an increase in anxiety and pain.

As a visitor it is possible for you to be involved in each of these interventions, but providing distraction is the most common contribution by friends and family members. For instance, conversation can decrease pain if the patient is alert. In addition, there are gifts you can give that may help to occupy the person's mind.

When the patient has been given a pain medication you should not expect the person to engage in coherent conversation. Most pain reducing drugs also have a sedating effect, making it more difficult for the person to think clearly and logically. Engaging such a patient in social conversation may be an unnecessary stress.

In addition to pain signaled by sensory nerves, a second kind of pain may occur. Brain originating pain can develop in persons who have been experiencing sensory pain. The discomfort resulting from tissue damage often causes patients to grimace, moan or complain about pain. When such behavior results in attention and special considerations that are not otherwise available, the brain can continue signaling the existence of pain even when there are no pain signals from the sensory nerves.

You can help to prevent such brain originating pain by keeping in mind two guidelines. First, in addition to supporting the patient when there is discomfort, be sure to pay attention to the person during periods of diminished pain. Second, allow the patient to engage in as much self-sufficient activity as is medically appropriate. By encouraging well behavior and by avoiding oversolicitious assistance, you can decrease the risk of brain originating pain.

A telephone call to the patient's room may be a way of gathering information relevant to the issues of embarrassment, current strength, need for sleep, and pain. As one former patient said, "I myself like to visit people in the hospital, but I make sure they are up to seeing people. I think it's best to call before you leave to see how the person sounds and feels."

If contact with the hospitalized individual is not possible, you may be able to communicate with a friend or relative in the room. When there is no one in the room who can provide information, another option is calling the nurses' station.

If the patient is able to talk on the phone, discussing when it will be convenient for you to drop by gives the person an opportunity to have some control over the situation. The hospital is a place where few people ask the patient's opinion about participating in activities. Instead, it is "Take a shower now," "I'm taking you to X ray" or "Here is your dinner." As one veteran patient told me, "When you give up your street clothes, you also give up a lot of freedom and control."

You can add some welcome self-control to the patient's life by allowing the person to participate in planning the timing of your visit. A previsit call also gives the patient an opportunity to look forward to your arrival.

In addition to providing a communication link for planning

visits, telephone calls themselves can be quite supportive. Here are the opinions of three patients.

- One of the most positive aspect of my hospital stay was "the telephone calls from my friends and loved ones."
- "I got a lot of phone calls from friends which helped a lot."
- "The flu was very prevalent at the time of my hospitalization, therefore many folks called on the telephone rather than visiting in-person, which was fine."

A telephone call can be an excellent idea if the patient is not up to a face-to-face encounter or if the hospital is too far away. In addition to these situations, another instance when a phone call is preferable to a visit is when you have contracted a communicable disease. You should not take a chance on giving your disease to others who already are sick.

Sending a message is a possibility if the patient is too ill for either a phone call or a visit. You can mail a note or a card, and, if the person has an audio tape player, you also have the option of sending a recorded message.

If it is decided that a visit is appropriate, there may need to be a decision about whether it is OK for a young family member to accompany you.

A visit by a child can be a positive experience for both the young visitor and the hospitalized individual. One patient enjoyed a visit from his two-and-one-half-year-old son who "told me new words he had learned." But visits by children also can be very unpleasant experiences for all concerned. One woman deeply regretted a visit she had made as a child: "It was thought my visit would cheer up my grandfather, but I was only four and I definitely made matters worse by crying and saying that wasn't my grandfather."

If the hospital allows young visitors, you should carefully consider the possible consequences before taking a child on a visit. You do not want to create unnecessary stress for either the child or the patient. But if you conclude that the young person will be able to handle both the patient's appearance and the hospital environment, then such a visit may be appropriate.

Demonstrating Respect During the Visit

Respect for the patient's needs should be your guiding principle during a hospital visit. Just as your planning ought to take into account the issues of embarrassment, strength, sleep and pain, you also should keep in mind the following considerations when you arrive at the hospital.

The nurses' station should be your first stop when you get to the patient's floor. Let them know whom you will be visiting, and ask if there are any special precautions necessary before entering the patient's room. Such restrictions may be for the sake of the person you are visiting or for the protection of other patients.

Whether or not a staff person mentions it, you should plan not to smoke during the visit. Even for patients who usually smoke themselves, inhaling tobacco smoke can be a very unpleasant experience for hospitalized individuals. In addition to patient discomfort, there also is an increased risk of fire if bottled oxygen is being used.

A hospital room doorway is the entrance to the patient's bedroom and bathroom. When you arrive at the person's room, you can further contribute to the individual's self-control by knocking if the door is closed.

A closed door often indicates the patient is being attended to by a staff member. Waiting for an answer to your knock can prevent your entrance at an inopportune moment.

Even if the door is open it still is appropriate to knock, although in such instances I often just say "knock, knock." This courtesy allows the patient an opportunity to invite you into the room. Wait for an invitation to enter if you would not go into the individual's bedroom without first being asked to come inside. If an invitation is appropriate but is not forthcoming, ask permission to come in and visit. The courtesy of waiting to be invited into the room gives control to the patient and allows for circumstances that may not be observable to you. For instance, a person about to use a bedpan may prefer that you delay your entrance for a few minutes.

Sometimes the patient may not be ready to receive the privacy you offer. Having become accustomed to the hospital routine, the patient may forget about being modest. For example, as a consulting psychologist in a small community hospital, I once visited a woman who greeted me, then threw back the sheet and got out of bed—wearing only a flimsy nightgown. I responded with a comment about needing to find a chair, as I turned away to look for one. Making my way to one of the room's two chairs, I suggested she put on her robe. She did, then we sat down and had a productive interaction. At times, you too may need to take the initiative in providing the patient with an appropriate amount of privacy.

Just as you should be willing to give the patient some privacy, you ought to be prepared to let a sleeping patient rest. If the person is taking a nap, it may be best for you to postpone your visit. You can check at the nurses' station about the advisability of awakening the patient. An OK from the staff gives you the freedom of deciding whether to awaken the person or to wait a bit longer.

Introducing yourself may be a good idea. Such an introduction is necessary for anyone standing outside a closed door, but it also may be appropriate even if the person can see you. For example, let's say the patient has been sleeping and has awakened just before your arrival. You know that when you wake up from a nap your mind may not immediately bring things into focus. This also is the case with hospitalized patients. In addition, medications, illness or pain can fog the person's thinking and perceiving. For all of these reasons, you should introduce yourself if there is any possibility that the person may not recognize who you are.

Your location with respect to the patient is important to consider. For instance, you may need think about your position with regard to lighting. You do not want to have a bright light at your back or to your side. Such an arrangement requires the patient to face a glare when looking at you, making it more difficult for the person to see your features and facial expressions. A situation you always should avoid is being between the patient and a sunlit window. Such positioning will strain the patient's eyes and will limit severely the person's ability to see you.

There are other considerations when selecting your location. You should be close enough to the patient so you can hear the person and so the patient can easily hear your voice. Your location also ought to be one that enables the individual to make eye contact with you without having to adopt an uncomfortable position. If there is more than one person visiting a patient, all of the visitors should be on the same side of the bed. When they are on opposite sides of the bed, the patient is forced to look back and forth—which can become very trying for the person.

Whether to stand or sit is a decision you will need to make. Standing may be a good choice if you intend on keeping your visit brief. Sitting implies you are going to stay awhile. For a patient in bed, it also means you are likely to be at eye level, rather than looking down on the person. So sitting may be your best choice if you want to communicate a willingness to stay and you wish to be on the same level as the patient.

If you decide to sit, the next question is where. Chairs often are in short supply in a hospital room. When a chair is available, you can move it to where eye contact with the patient is the most comfortable. (Be sure to return the chair to its original location before you leave.) If you wish to sit, but there is no chair available, a logical alternative is to sit on the patient's bed.

Sitting on the bed is a good option if you can answer yes to each of the following statements.

- ☐ You have sat on the patient's bed at home.
- ☐ You wish to look down on the patient (sitting on the bed usually means your head will be above the patient's).
- ☐ The staff approves.

Sitting on the person's bed is an intimate behavior that usually should be avoided. But there is another intimate behavior that often is appropriate.

Touch may be an important channel of communication for you to use. It can convey warmth, caring and support. Unfortuantely, many friends and family members shy away from touching patients. For example, in one study of breast cancer patients, half of the women reported that others avoided physical contact.

Touching the patient provides helpful support if the following criteria are met.

- [ ] It is appropriate for the circumstances. For instance, the patient's condition is not contagious.
- [ ] It communicates an acceptable level of intimacy. Many of our natural inhibitions against touch fall away during health crises. But touch can be a very personal way of interacting, and some patients remain uncomfortable with such intimacy.
- [ ] It conveys positive messages such as caring and acceptance rather than negative messages such as condescension or dominance.
- [ ] It is not painful. Surgery, IV's, other treatments or the patient's condition can make the person more sensitive to painful stimulation. Be aware of these possibilities when you think about touching the patient. For instance, one gravely ill patient would ask visitors to hold her hand. But when the visitor offered a hand she would say "Don't hold mine, let me hold yours, because your hand is too heavy." She wanted the comfort of the physical contact, but she knew she had to beware of the pain it could cause.

Controlled research demonstrates that touch decreases anxiety when the hospital patient appreciates such contact. But the same research also shows that touch increases anxiety if the patient is uncomfortable with physical contact.

If you touch the person, be alert for the individual's reactions. A good indication of acceptance is reciprocal touch by the patient. But if the patient does not seek to return your touch or if touching seems to make the person feel uncomfortable, then abandon physical contact in favor of words and jestures.

Conversations always should respect the patient's needs. For instance, when there are two or more visitors in the room be sure to give the patient an opportunity to participate in any interaction. One patient told me that the worst part of having visits was that "sometimes a group of visitors would carry on a conversation without me" and another complained that "visitors talk to each other and forget to talk to [the] patient." If you wish to exclude the patient from a conversation you should choose another time and place for that discussion.

Sometimes a medical professional may check on the patient while you are with the person, and you may think of something you want to ask about the patient's condition. If this happens, first ask yourself if it is necessary and appropriate for you to know the answer. A "yes" to this question should be followed by considering the possibility of first asking the patient. If the patient doesn't know the answer, it may be more appropriate for the patient to ask the question than for you to ask it.

The one action you should not take is to follow the professional out of the room in order to talk with the staff member. Such an incident may cause the patient to wonder what it is that you don't want to be heard. The person may begin to question how straightforward you are being or whether things are much worse than what others have said.

Trust in the staff is another patient need you should respect during conversation. If you make negative comments about the nurses or doctors you may undermine the patient's confidence in the medical personnel.

As mentioned earlier, dissatisfaction with the staff is the most common patient complaint. If the individual describes a difficulty with the staff it is appropriate to reflect the person's concern (Chapter 3) and to involve the patient in problem solving (Chapter 2), but you should think twice before engaging in criticism yourself. Critical comments on your part only serve to weaken the patient's belief in the staff—unless you intend to do something about the problem you perceive. If you do decide to express a concern to the staff, your opinions should be communicated in ways that are consistent with the staff interaction guidelines discussed in the next chapter.

Staying an Appropriate Length of Time

- "Many [visitors] stayed too long for my comfort."
- The most negative aspect of my hospital stay was "visitors staying too long."
- Visits are "very tiring at times. [I appreciate] shorter but more frequent visits."
- "Sometimes [visitors] stayed too long when I was tired. It got kind of boring when we ran out of things to say and they felt they had to stay."
- "Some stayed too long for me to have enough time with my husband."
- "I do believe hospital visits should be short—usually no more than 30 minutes."
- I thought 30- to 60-minute "visits were too long and tiring."
- "I would like my family and friends to visit, staying only a half hour at a time."
- I would like to be visited by "my close friends, but not to stay over 15 minutes."
- "Fifteen minutes is long enough for visits when the patient is not feeling well."
- "I believe shorter visits are less tiring."

A friend of mine recently had her second child, two-and-one-half years after having her first. Both daughters were born in the same hospital, but the maternity visiting hours radically changed between her first and second deliveries. During her first stay in the maternity ward, visitors were allowed on the unit for a total of one hour per day. But by her second delivery, visiting hours had been expanded to 12 hours per day. She said that during those 12 hours she rarely had a moment to herself. It was too much of a good thing. By the end of her hospital stay she felt exhausted and in need of a rest.

Visitors staying too long is the most common complaint that patients have about family and friends. If you are providing the advocacy support discussed in Chapter 2, then long visits can be appropriate. Otherwise, long visits may have the following negative effects.

- [ ] As demonstrated by the preceding patient quotes, overly long visits can be tiring and boring. They also can rob the patient of time to be with close family members.
- [ ] Paradoxically, an overly long visit can decrease the patient's willingness to seek support from you. Such a visit emphasizes the sacrifice you are making on behalf of the patient. Having seen the trouble to which you have gone, the person may feel a strong sense of indebtedness. Once feeling indebted, the individual can become hesitant to ask for any further help from you.

Rather than demonstrating your concern by staying a long time, it may be more important for the patient to know that you are a reliable source of support. Staying for a reasonable amount of time and offering further support is a better strategy than an overly long visit.

But what is an appropriate length for a hospital visit? Certainly there are differences among patients, as well as changes from one visit to the next for the same patient.

I know one minister who believes a sure sign that he has stayed long enough is when a patient says "I'm so glad you came" or "I really appreciate your visit." If you receive such a comment after the first few minutes of your visit, you too may want to consider whether it is time to go.

Recognizing that patients' needs vary, the most common maximum visit lengths that patients mention are between 15 and 30 minutes.

If you intend to visit the patient for a certain amount of time, you still should be flexible enough to modify your plans based upon the changing conditions and the needs of the person. There are two common situations that require such flexibility.

☐ You should be sensitive to the patient's need for therapeutic and evaluation procedures. For example, if the physical therapy aide comes for the patient, your visit should not delay the session.

☐ You also should pay attention to how many visitors are in the room. Most hospitals have rules on the number of visitors allowed per patient. As a visitor, you share the responsibility of ensuring that the number of people in the room remains at an appropriate level. This may mean delaying your visit or cutting it short in favor of new visitors.

Here is the response of one former patient when asked to describe her thoughts about visiting hospitalized individuals.

- "I feel as though I should know the patient closely, for he may be embarrassed or uncomfortable otherwise. Also, I try to gauge the length of the visit according to his strength and level of recuperation. Visits are cheering in-person because loneliness and boredom may result without them. I don't like to interfere in any way with the medical treatment and nurses and doctors. Whenever the patient has to be treated, I leave the room....To show the patient that I care about him is my main goal....[The most positive aspect of visiting an individual in the hospital is] to see some improvement in the patient's psychological well-being and to know I have made him happy for a short while."

If you have similar attitudes to those expressed by this individual, it will be easy to implement the hospital visit etiquette described in this chapter.

5

The Patient's Medical Family

When I asked patients to describe the best part of being in the hospital, the most frequent reply was the care from the staff.

- "The nursing staff and doctor treated me with excellent care."
- "The medical and nursing staffs were very knowledgeable and attentive."
- The best aspect of being hospitalized was "the excellent care from the nursing staff and from my doctor."
- The best part of being in the hospital was "the care and attention that I received from the nursing staff."
- "The nurses showed a lot of concern and care for me."
- The most positive aspect of my hospital stay was "the way that the doctors were straightforward with me and would answer any questions I had—they didn't try to hide anything."
- The best part of my hospitalization was "that my doctor would come in to examine me, but he was never in a hurry. He'd always explain any questions and everything he was going to do in language you would understand."

- The best aspect of being in the hospital was "the thoughtful manner in which my family and I were prepared for each new procedure by the staff."
- The most positive aspect of being in the hospital was "prompt service from nursing staff making me feel comfortable and easily relaxed."
- I really appreciated "the care of the nursing staff when I was in a great deal of pain. The nurses listened and did not make me feel guilty when I complained."
- The best part of being in the hospital was the "excellent treatment by staff in the ICU [and] concern shown for the patient. Kind nurses [were] always ready to give me what was needed."
- The most postive aspect of my hospital stay was "physical therapy. The people there were fantastic. The aides that transported me there were very uplifting. It really helped my morale."
- "Friendly nurses brightened the stay."
- The best part of being hospitalized was "the high level of care and attention which I received from all members of the hospital staff."
- I really liked "the friendliness of the entire hospital staff. The nurses kept your spirits up. They gave me a lift when I needed it most."

I also asked patients to identify the most negative aspect of being in the hospital. The most frequent response was problems with the staff.

- "I would like the medical staff to be more honest with me.... I never knew how they felt about my sickness or what they were planning on doing."
- "I think patients should be told exactly what medications they are being given and why. I was put on Valium® to avoid spasms. I would have preferred the spasms."
- "The doctor always was in a hurry. Sometimes we need to ask questions and we want answers."
- "The hospital staff had little time to talk to me and explain things."

- "My doctor seemed to treat me more as a 'guinea pig' than a person and was very illusive with me."
- "Doctors left me alone for about half an hour in the operating room after surgery. No one told me what was going on....I'd like to be told more about what they were doing to me."
- The most negative aspect of my hospital stay was "the way the nurses took so long to give me pain pills and the way they complained and tried to tell me I wasn't in as much pain as I said."
- "When you ask for a pain shot—they tell you they'll bring it right in—then you wait for an hour. If it isn't time they should just tell you it's not time."
- "The nurses were slow and didn't care about getting your medication."
- I did not like "some of the surgeon's assistants and other doctors called in for consultation. They didn't listen and [were] in too much of a hurry."

Just as there are difficulties within an extended family from time to time, problems sometimes develop between the patient and medical personnel. Before considering what to do when difficulties occur, let's examine the roles and responsibilities within the patient's medical family.

The Medical Family Tree

The attending physician is the doctor who is responsible for supervising the patient's case. (Often this is the physician who admitted the patient to the hospital, although the admitting doctor may be someone else.) Much of the attending physician's supervision takes place by means of the patient's medical chart—the doctor writes orders in the chart that are to be carried out by other members of the hospital staff. Some of the most important orders are written to the nursing staff.

These directives include how often the patient is to be observed, what kinds of observations are to be made, what physical activities are allowed and what drugs are to be administered.

In addition to using the chart to give orders, the doctor also uses it to receive information about the patient. For example, the nurses write their observations in the chart and note the administration of any drugs or other ordered care.

Often the attending physician will request consultation from another medical speciality. For instance, if the doctor orders a radiological consult, X rays will be taken and the radiologist's report will be placed in the patient's chart. Such consults by other doctors are very common, but it is the attending physician who is ultimately responsible for using consultation information to plan the patient's care.

The medical specialties available will depend upon the size and mission of the hospital. In addition to radiology, other commonly found specialties include the following:

anesthesiology (therapeutic loss of sensation)
cardiology (heart)
dentistry (teeth, jaws and mouth)
dermatology (skin)
emergency medicine (you name it)
endocrinology (metabolic disturbances affecting the thyroid, pancreas or other endocrine glands)
family medicine (traditionally medicine's front line in the community)
gastroenterology (stomach and intestines)
hematology (blood)
oncology (cancer)

internal medicine (includes infectious disease as well as the following specialties: cardiology, endocrinology, gastroenterology, hematology, oncology, nephrology, pulmonary medicine, rheumatology)
nephrology (kidneys)
neurology (brain and nervous system)
obstetrics/gynecology (bringing life into the world and functions associated with that talent)
ophthalmology (eyes)
orthopedics (bones and joints)
otolaryngology (ears, nose and throat)
pathology (disease investigation)
pediatrics (infants and children)
psychiatry (brain and behavior)
pulmonary medicine (lungs)
rheumatology (muscles and joints)
urology (urinary tract and male reproductive system)
general surgery (generic operations)
cardiovascular and thoracic surgery (heart, lungs and nearby areas)
colon and rectal surgery (operations at the end of the line)
oral and maxillofacial surgery (mouth, jaws and face).

Each medical speciality is supervised by a department chief, who is responsible for the quality of care offered by the physicians on the staff in that unit. If the hospital provides physician training there may be additional individuals on the department staff. *Fourth year medical students* (also called *interns*) may have limited patient responsibilities. *Residents* have completed their four-year medical degrees and are specializing within the particular area of medicine represented by the department. Chief or senior residents are in their last year of residency with the department.

In addition to coordinating care, attending physicians apply their own diagnostic and therapeutic skills. This involves making regular observations of their patients. It is during such contacts that the patient normally can ask the doctor questions or express concerns.

But what if the patient's attending physician is replaced by another doctor. Often this means the attending physician is off for the day and the replacement is temporary. Sometimes though, there will be a change in the physician responsible for the patient's care and a new doctor will become the attending physician. Such a switch is most likely when the nature of the patient's condition changes. For example, a patient hospitalized for an appendectomy develops heart problems, and the surgeon who removed the appendix transfers the case to a heart specialist. The change is noted on the patient's chart and the hospital staff is made aware of the transfer.

Sometimes the patient will be moved to a new room where specialized care is more readily available. The explanation of such a room change is likely to include the fact that there also is a new attending physician.

For one reason or another, there are rare instances in which a patient is not told of a change in doctors. Usually such an occurrence represents an accidental failure in communication. The staff intends to let the patient know what is happening, but the information about the switch doesn't get communicated. For example, there is a change in attending physicians, but the patient stays in the same room, and the original doctor continues to visit, although a new doctor also sees the patient each afternoon. From the patient's perspective it may seem as though little has changed, and the person is not likely to know about the shift in medical responsibility unless a staff member provides information about the switch.

In most instances the involvement of additional doctors in a case does not mean there is a new attending physician. Usually the other doctors are acting as consultants or are temporary replacements. But if a different physician stops by, it is appropriate to clarify the new doctor's role and to confirm who has the attending physician responsibilities.

Nursing staff members usually are the personnel who have the most contact with the patient. *Registered nurses* (RN's) will monitor the patient's status and see to it that prescribed care is provided. Should medical difficulties arise, it probably will be an RN who first analyzes the situation and who decides upon the initial response to the new developments.

While nurses provide general patient care on medical floors, there also are specialized nursing services. For instance, operating rooms and recovery rooms have their own specially trained nursing staffs.

Registered nurses usually are assisted by two kinds of support staff. *Licensed practical nurses* (LPN's) often provide much of the care that is considered routine in nature. *Attendants*, *aides* and *orderlies* may provide fundamental care such as giving baths, changing the linen and bringing drinks.

Sometimes it may be difficult to determine the job classification of a staff member without looking at the person's name tag. But each position has its own set of responsibilities and its own educational requirements.

An RN has passed a state-administered examination and is certified to practice nursing. Some registered nurses have two-year college degrees and others have two- or three-year degrees from hospital-based nursing programs. More and more registered nurses now have four-year degrees, and many have masters degrees in nursing.

An LPN has a one-year degree from a program in practical nursing. Some staff members may be *vocational nurses* who have graduated from a high school program in practical nursing.

Attendants, aides and orderlies receive their training while on the job. The sophistication of the care they provide depends upon the level to which they have progressed.

Registered nurses are the professionals who are responsible for the day-to-day operation of the unit. An RN develops a nursing care plan for each patient, and registered nurses continue to be responsible for seeing that the plan is implemented. A *charge nurse* supervises the registered nurses and staff assistants serving on the shift.

(The three most common shifts are: day shift - 7:00 a.m. to 3:30 p.m.; evening shift - 3:00 p.m. to 11:30 p.m.; night shift - 11:00 p.m. to 7:30 a.m. Nurses are very busy during the shift overlap times—usually 3:00 to 3:30 p.m., 11:00 to 11:30 p.m., and 7:00 to 7:30 a.m. The outgoing shift gives a report to the incoming shift and there is much to be covered. When possible, it is better to interact with nurses at times other than the change of shift.)

Some hospitals have two other kinds of nursing positions—head nurse and primary nurse. A *head nurse*, or *nursing coordinator*, is responsible for all three shifts on a unit. The head nurse's hours often overlap the day and evening shifts. In addition to the position of head nurse, some hospitals also have a system of primary care nursing. If this is the case, a *primary care nurse* will be responsible for the nursing care of a patient in much the same way the that the attending physician is responsible for physician-directed care. The primary care nurse develops the patient's nursing care plan, provides much of that care and arranges other needed services.

The *director of nursing* is the administrator responsible for the nursing component of the hospital. As with head nurses, the director's workday usually overlaps the first and second shifts.

Other staff members, in addition to the medical and nursing staffs, are associated with a number of service components within the hospital. These may include admissions, business operations, chaplin's office, dietary services, housekeeping, maintenance, medical records, occupational therapy, patient education, patient representative services, physical therapy, recreational therapy, respiratory therapy, social services, speech and hearing, and volunteer services.

Interacting With the Staff

A need for information is commonly felt by both patients and visitors. For instance, there usually is a strong need to know the patient's status; this includes knowing what outcome is expected (the prognosis) and understanding the nature of the medical services being provided. It also means wanting to be informed when there is a major change in the prognosis or in the services received by the patient.

Frequently there are changes in a patient's treatment. Most of these changes are planned, but there are rare instances in which care is offered to one patient when it actually is intended for another person. Examples include medication, meals, physical therapy, and—in the extreme—surgery. When a form of care is offered that is unexpected, it is valid to question its appropriateness. If a staff member persists in offering a service that does not seem to make sense, one can request that the attending physician be consulted before the change is implemented.

Here are some relevant comments by a veteran patient. "I have had positive hospital experiences but I still feel that I should check on or oversee medications/treatments that are given to me—some mistakes have been made in communication between M.D.'s and nurses. A patient should strive to be well-informed about what his physician will do. You should ask questions before hospitalization, so that you know what will be required of you and the nursing staff. They change every 8 hours and sometimes continuity of medical care depends on you. Speak up if something doesn't seem right. Make the nurses check with the M.D. if necessary. Sometimes they have misread the orders."

If you need to know about the patient's condition or treatment, it may be best to ask the hospitalized individual first. (But remember not to be an interrogator.) Often the patient will have the information you desire. When it is not possible to ask the patient, it may appropriate for an immediate family member or close friend to seek information from the medical or nursing staff.

Requesting information from the staff is one appropriate way of interacting with the patient's medical family. But there also may be times when you can provide valuable input regarding the patient's care.

Serving as a patient's advocate, as discussed in Chapter 2, can be an important form of support by a friend or family member. Often a patient's ability to communicate is diminished during a hospital stay. Illness, surgical procedures or drugs can interfere with the person's ability to articulate questions and concerns. If this occurs, an advocate may be able to help the staff better understand the patient's status so that appropriate services are provided.

Just before I wrote the preceding sentences I found a note I had written to my wife while I was hospitalized for throat surgery. It reads, "They gave me a shot for pain this morning—it didn't help much. Nothing since then. Would you see if I can have a pain pill?"

Now why would I write such a note to my wife instead of communicating with one of the nurses myself? Well, for one thing, it was only a few hours since the surgery and talking was painful. Also, the shot I had been given seemed to telescope my perception of time. I remember thinking that the nurses appeared to move like hummingbirds—one instant a nurse would be in the room and the next instant she would be gone. But for whatever reason, I had failed to notify the staff of my pain, and I had not requested additional medication. After receiving the note, my wife went to the nurses' station and a few minutes later a nurse brought me some pain medication.

My experience with the pain shot is not uncommon. Although a drug may be expected to have a certain therapeutic benefit, a given medication may not have the desired effect for a particular patient. The staff needs to know if this occurs or if there are undesired side effects. As my wife did for me, it may be appropriate for you to inform the staff of the patient's condition. Once they know about unwanted effects, they can make appropriate adjustments in the kind or amount of medication.

There are other situations in which an advocate can help the patient to communicate with the hospital staff. For example, patients sometimes are confused about the reasons for tubes and lines connected to their bodies. Instead of asking a doctor or nurse, the patient may feel more at ease communicating a question to you.

If the patient does ask you a medical question, first try to get a good understanding of what is on the person's mind. Use reflection to summarize your perception of the concern and the feelings associated with it. Once you believe you have covered the important points, find out what the patient wants done. Maybe the person now feels ready to communicate the concern to the staff. Or maybe it will be appropriate for you to act as a messenger and talk to a staff member on behalf of the patient. But before choosing the latter option, double-check with the person to make sure you are being asked to speak to the staff.

There are rare instances in which it is appropriate for an advocate to disagree with those in authority. For instance, a friend of mine recently gave birth to a baby and the staff used a new procedure during her labor. After having the baby she became nauseated and was unable to keep anything down. Her doctor put her on an IV and told her the nausea was a temporary reaction to the new procedure he had used.

As the nausea persisted her condition worsened, but the physician stuck by his diagnosis and made no changes in his orders for her. After she had been in the hospital for a week, her father paid a visit and was appalled at her condition. He demanded that she be evaluated by another doctor and a surgeon was called to examine her. Within 15 minutes she was in an operating room; a section of intestine had become twisted and was blocking her digestive system. If the surgery had not taken place when it did, it is possible that she would have died. My friend's father may have helped to save her life by disagreeing with the attending physician.

What would you have done if you had been the parent of my friend?

Studies show that visitors and patients often question various aspects of the hospital experience but don't communicate their concerns because they believe that good hospital behavior is to be quiet, passive and accepting. This reluctance to express dissatisfaction is understandable, since the patient's dependence upon the staff can result in a fear of displeasing the doctors and nurses. But such passivity can prevent important exchanges of information.

On the other hand, some visitors are too quick to be critical of the staff. One nurse told me the following story. "I had a lady die one evening during visiting hours. I stayed with her and her family through to the end—holding her hand and her family's. After she had died I left the room, with tears in my eyes, to go tell her doctor. I was confronted by a lady at the nurses' station wanting to know where I'd been and why hadn't her father gotten his evening cigarette yet. When I'd explained that I'd been with a very ill patient she responded with 'You nurses always have some excuse why you're not doing what you're supposed to be doing.' At times I think a lot of visitors have this same attitude. I hope not because most of us nurses really do care and attitudes like that make it harder when we ask ourselves why we do this."

Neither passivity nor hostility are appropriate ways of handling opinions you have that differ from those of the staff. Instead, it is possible to disagree in ways that are likely to result in mutual understanding and suitable action.

Assertive communication is an appropriate way to express disagreement. You can effectively communicate an opposing point of view if you prepare yourself in two ways and then follow five guidelines as you interact with the staff member.

Here are the two preparations.

- ☐ **Remember your purpose** is to foster proper patient care—a goal that both you and the staff share.
- ☐ **Plan ahead.** Most nurses and physicians have a multitude of responsibilities. When you talk with those in authority,

it often is a brief encounter. Make the most of the interaction by organizing your thoughts ahead of time. If you have several topics to discuss it may be helpful to make a list of concerns.

Once you are face-to-face with a staff member, remember your purpose and plan as you implement the following five guidelines.

- **Avoid talking in front of an audience** if you believe it is necessary to confront a staff member on a particular issue. When you are free from direct observation by others, both of you may feel more willing to speak openly, thereby enhancing the possibility of a positive outcome. (Do not talk with a staff member just outside of the patient's earshot. It can be very anxiety provoking to know that others are discussing one's case while being unable to discern what they are saying.)
- **Be direct and honest** in stating what is on your mind. For example, let's say you notice a nurse bringing a new medication and you are concerned that it might be the wrong medicine. You could say, "Why are you giving that medicine?" But "why" questions often are perceived as threats, and they tend to put the other person on the defensive.

   When you question a staff member's actions, it is better to state your opinion about the situation and then say what you would like to happen or what you want to know. For instance, you might say "This seems to be a new medication. I would appreciate it if you would check on the reason for the change." Phrasing your input in this way is more likely to generate positive results than a "why" question or other indirect accusation.

- ☐ **Describe a specific situation** that gave rise to concern. For example, "This morning you said you would be right in with a pain shot, but it was an hour before you brought it." Avoid vague generalities, such as "You never listen," and do not make attributions about motivation, such as "You don't care about getting medication." Generalizations and comments on perceived personality traits tend to sidetrack interactions, whereas specific descriptions of events are more likely to focus attention on the issues in need of clarification or change.
- ☐ **Display nonverbal behavior that is consistent** with your words. This includes standing erect, regularly making eye contact with the person as you talk, and speaking in a normal conversational tone of voice. Try to avoid expressing irritation unintentionally through your tone of voice, posture or facial expressions.
- ☐ **Reflect responses** by the staff member. This will ensure that you are understanding the person. Reflection also helps in handling any anger you may feel during the conversation. When you first reflect before responding with your own opinion, it slows the interaction and helps you to stay in control.

If you follow these suggestions the other person is likely to understand what is on your mind. Once the staff member accurately perceives your concern, the person is more likely to provide an appropriate explanation or institute proper action.

You now have read about issues concerning support, communication, etiquette, and the staff that relate to hospital patients in general. But some circumstances require additional considerations. The next chapter examines six special situations.

6

Special Considerations

- "It was traumatic to leave my parents....It might be helpful that others know what [a child is] experiencing" (comments from an adult recalling a childhood hospitalization).
- "The intensive care unit [was] very depressing."
- Visiting my aunt in the psychiatric unit "makes me feel sad and helpless."
- My father was in a "severe car accident. We couldn't talk. He lost his coordination due to brain damage, so his speech was very slow and slurred together."
- "The most awkward aspect [of visiting a patient like my aunt who had terminal cancer] is the total lack of knowing what to say. The situation is so serious that somehow, words provide very little it seems. The worst part is definitely the feeling of imminent loss."
- I visited my mother 9 or 10 times after her car accident, then she died. "Because of her death, I avoid the hospital as much as possible."

Each of these situations requires special considerations in addition to the material you have read in the preceding chapters. Consequently, this chapter examines needs associated with hospitalized children, patients in special care units,

Children

- "I was very frightened."
- The most negative part of my hospital stay was "not knowing anyone."

Helping the patient to maintain a sense of permanence is one benefit of any interaction with a hospitalized friend or relative. Your contact is a tangible reminder that certain aspects of life remain stable and durable, even through tumultuous events such as hospitalization and illness. The idea of permanence is especially important for children, and continued identification with one's home has been shown to be a major contributor to childhood health.

During times of uncertainty and stress, there is a basic need for things that are familiar. Adult patients often like to have their own pillows and other personal articles. Items from home are even more important for children. A favorite stuffed animal, special toys or other reminders of home can be comforting to the young patient.

If you help the child with daily self-care tasks at home, having your familiar presence takes some of the strangeness out of similar tasks at the hospital. The young person may appreciate your assistance when it is time to eat, bathe or use the toilet. Helping with such routine activities is a concrete way of demonstrating the bond that continues between the two of you.

Should you decide to lend a hand, be sure what you are doing is consistent with the medical regimen being provided to the child. If you have any doubts about the appropriateness of your assistance, check with a nurse or the attending physician.

Objects play an important role in the young patient's world because of the child's concrete style of thinking. Rather than sitting and talking, it often is a good idea to center the interaction on a game or toy. Ironically, talking with a child often becomes easier when conversation is seen as incidental to the ongoing activity. If you bring a game, a puzzle or some other toy, the gift can become the focus of your visit.

(As with task assistance, be sure any gift you give is appropriate. Consider both the child's age and medical condition. For instance, do not bring marbles for a three-year-old who might swallow them, and avoid giving barrettes to a girl who is losing her hair due to chemotherapy.)

Games that are magnetic or electronic in nature can be fun and are easy to use in bed. For example, devices such as portable video games or magnetic checkers can be enjoyable.

While you are with the child, a number of activities outside of the room may be possible. For instance, a wheelchair ride can be a fun experience if the child is up to it and the staff agree. Slow walks are another possibility if the young patient is ambulatory. Some hospitals have playrooms for their pediatric patients.

Children often want to know what is happening at school, at home and in the neighborhood. Information you can provide about life on the outside is likely to be of interest to the patient.

For some children, one appreciated reminder from home can be a visit from a special pet. There are hospitals that encourage pet visits and make arrangements for them when possible.

Activities that allow children to express their thoughts and emotions in concrete ways may be especially helpful. Such items include puppets, dolls, "action figures," stuffed animals, art supplies, writing materials, construction toys and craft kits. Self-expression through these kinds of activities often allows a child the opportunity to share perceptions and questions that otherwise might be difficult or impossible for the young person to communicate.

For example, a ten-year-old tonsillectomy patient felt "the staff of the hospital was very unsympathetic," but he kept his feelings to himself. Looking back on his hospitalization years later, he observed, "I was young and [too afraid] to ask questions."

Through play activities a child may communicate similar kinds of fears to you. Let's say you are visiting a five-year-old girl. She pretends that her doll asks the nurse a question and that the nurse spanks the doll for asking. Such a pretend scenario may result from the same sort of concerns kept hidden by the young tonsillectomy patient.

Your best response is to first recognize that being afraid to ask questions is understandable. Then you might have the doll ask the question again (in a polite way). This time have the pretend nurse give an appropriate and realistic answer.

After addressing the issue in play, you might say to the child "I get the feeling you would like to ask the nurse a question." Often the young person will open up at that point. If not, you might say "If you were going to ask the nurse a question, what would it be?"

Once the child has told you what is on her mind, offer to have the nurse come into the room so the patient actually can ask the question. If the young person is reluctant, assure her that you will be there when she asks. In most cases this kind of encouragement will be sufficient to get the child to express her concerns and test their legitimacy.

Should the patient open up with you further, remember that

your best initial response probably is reflection. The communication skills discussed in Chapter 3 are especially applicable when visiting a child.

Although two-way communication is important, there may be times when the child will be perfectly happy to have the bulk of the activity come from you. For example, your reading of a story can become a highlight of the child's day. Even older children may like to have stories read to them. For instance, one woman told me about being hospitalized when she was eleven. She recalled that having "my mother read to me" was one of the memorable aspects of her hospitalization.

If the young person has a cassette recorder—a good gift idea if the child doesn't have one—you may want to record your rendition of a story so the patient can hear it again at another time. A cassette recorder (preferably with earphones) also makes it possible for the child to listen to a variety of books and stories that are commercially available on tape. Listening to such material can help the child to pass the time when you and others are not available.

Activity on your part can be important even if the child is unable to respond. When a young person is very ill or semiconscious there may be little or no reaction to you. Although there may be no acknowledgment of you, the child still may be aware of your presence.

Your touch and voice may help the patient remain oriented. The simple act of holding the child's hand can communicate a great deal of love and reassurance. And hearing a familiar voice can be especially comforting.

If you tire of carrying on a one-way conversation, you can read from a book or magazine. It probably does not matter very much what you read to an unresponsive child; the importance is in the fact that you are providing a familiar voice that may reach the young person.

Don't burden the child with your problems. Take time to compose yourself if you have had a tough day or a difficult time getting to the hospital. It is better to take a break than to rush into the room and appear distracted by other concerns. (You might want to try some of the stress management techniques described in Chapter 7.) Even if this has not been one of your better days, you can take control and prepare yourself for a productive visit.

Avoid blaming the child for the hospitalization. Such confrontations—even when accurate—serve no useful purpose while the child is in the hospital. They only weaken the potential positive effects of your visit.

Distorting or denying the reality of the situation is another way of risking one's relationship with a hospitalized child. Should your statements turn out not to be true, the patient may come to believe you are not to be trusted.

It is tempting to hide the painfulness of a procedure from a child or to deny the seriousness of a grave condition. But the young patient will feel betrayed if experience shows that things really are very different from what you have indicated. Such a child is likely to remain mistrustful and suspicious. Having been robbed of an important relationship, the patient may be more vulnerable to the stresses of hospitalization.

The ending of your visit is one important issue about which you should be honest. The child may be sad to see you go and may cry.

Some visitors sneak out in order to avoid seeing the young person unhappy. This tactic is easy on the visitor but very rough on the child. During the next visit the patient is likely to be anxious—realizing that the person could leave at any moment. Consequently, rather than being a calming influence, the visit can turn into a stressful episode for the child.

It is much better for you to give clear cues that your visit is about to end and to tell the child that it is time for you to go. There still may be sadness and crying, but during your next visit the patient will not be worrying constantly about when you are going to leave. If possible, tell the young person when you expect to return. (As you go out, also leave this information at the nurses' station.) Knowing when your next visit is planned gives the child a concrete event to anticipate. Looking forward to that time can provide something to hope for that will be realized in the short-term.

Spending the night with a child is an option available for parents in most hospitals. In some areas, this opportunity is mandated by law. For instance, in Canada parents have the legal right to visit their hospitalized child at any time and to participate in the patient's care. Some states have similar regulations. For example, in Massachusetts the parents of a hospitalized child are given the right of "constant parental support of and contact with the pediatric patient throughout hospitalization."

Even if there is no formal sleep-over program, those in authority may be able to allow such arrangements. Should your first request be met with a denial, check with the attending physician and ask for a note suggesting permission for your overnight stay. Such a request from the child's doctor is likely to carry quite a bit of weight in the decision-making process.

Most medical professionals recognize that rooming-in can be a valuable contributor to a child's well-being. For example, one nurse told me about the hospitalizations of her five-year-old son and her four-year-old daughter. Rooming-in was possible with her daughter and she remained with the child throughout the brief hospitalization. She chose to stay in order "to provide support and a sense of security."

This nurse's concern is well-founded. For instance, another woman described to me her hospitalization as a six-year-old. She recalled that "It was traumatic to leave (my) parents," and that her separation from them was the most negative aspect of being in the hospital.

Research involving three- to six-year-old patients consistently shows positive effects when a parent rooms in with the child. Such parental availablilty appears to be most important during periods of high stress.

One high-stress time is the child's first night in the hospital. For instance, my wife recalls that this was the scariest part of her childhood hospitalization; unfortunately, parental rooming-in was not allowed at that time. But most hospitals have changed their policies since then. Medical professionals now recognize that the security of a nearby parent can greatly ease a young person's fears. Although the visitor's bed may not be elegant, spending the night with the patient should be considered for any newly hospitalized child.

Having a parent or other close relative with the child at the beginning of the hospitalization can provide both moral and decision-making support. Not only is it reassuring to the patient, but the presence of such a person can improve the flow of communication between the child and the staff. A knowledgeable visitor may be able to help others more accurately perceive the young patient's needs.

If you are familiar with the child's usual behavior and temperament, you have a standard from which to judge the severity of any complaints or difficulties. Consequently, your observations and interpretations of the patient's behavior can be helpful to the staff. If you perceive a change in the child's behavior it may be important for the staff to know your impressions, since you may be able to judge the degree of change taking place. For instance, if you are accustomed to how the child expresses pain, you are in an excellent position to evaluate the severity of the young person's discomfort. Informing the staff when the patient needs pain medication is one example of how you can use your knowledge of the child to foster good medical care.

Keeping tabs on the child's status does not require a constant flow of questions on your part. One woman, recalling an illness when she was thirteen, remembered how comforting and reassuring it was to have her mother in the room. But at the same time, she recalled being irritated because her mother kept asking questions about how she was doing. Such continuous interrogation is not necessary in order to effectively monitor a young patient.

If you do decide to room in, plan to take some breaks. Should you believe constant companionship is necessary, arrange for your spouse or another trusted adult to fill in for you. Use the time to get something to eat, take a walk, or run errands. You will find that allowing yourself such breaks will better enable you to handle the demands of providing support for the child.

In some hospitals there are rooms set aside for use by families of patients who are having prolonged hospitalizations. Other hospitals have a Ronald McDonald House or similar facility nearby that provides housing for the families of hospitalized children. Should you or someone you know require such assistance, check with the hospital's social service department for the necessary information.

The need for a familiar adult's presence tends to decrease as the hospitalization progresses. With time, the strangeness of the hospital subsides and the child becomes more accustomed to the daily routine. And just as the patient becomes more used to the setting, staff members become more familiar with the patient and are better able to understand the young person.

You will need to monitor the situation and judge how long your visits should be. The average parent spends five hours a day with a hospitalized child, but there is tremendous variation. One of the sources of variation is the length of the child's stay in the hospital. Parents of chronically ill children tend to become more selective in their visiting time—usually staying the longest on important days involving events such as admission, surgery, major procedures or tests, and discharge. These veterans know that on a surgery day it is good for a parent to be with the child before the operation—which may involve spending the night or arriving very early in the morning. It also is advisable to be present as the young patient regains consciousness, when the comforting touch and voice of a familiar adult can be very reassuring.

Wondering what is causing their symptoms is a natural reaction for patients. Adults usually think about the possible nature of their physical problem, but preschool children often do not connect their symptoms to a physical malfunction. Instead, they frequently see their condition as the result of some misbehavior on their part. A three-year-old boy in pain may interpret his discomfort as punishment for one of his misdeeds. Even up to ages eight or ten, children tend to look to events of the recent past to explain their predicament. For example, a nine-year-old girl may believe she became sick because she disobeyed her mother.

Often children keep such beliefs to themselves rather than sharing their thoughts with others. When kept inside, such distorted interpretations tend to become more firmly entrenched and less amenable to change. In order to get their concerns out in the open, children need others in whom to confide. They need to be able to share their feelings and to test the accuracy of their beliefs.

Common concerns for young patients include: being separated from parents, peers, and one's usual routines; being afraid of strangers and of unfamiliar surroundings; dread of anticipated procedures; and pain or discomfort during medical interventions.

It is not necessarily a bad sign for a child to cry or become depressed as an initial response to a difficult situation. Having openly expressed their emotions, such children often are able to tolerate stressful procedures better than those who keep their feelings inside.

Children are very perceptive, a fact adults sometimes forget. For example, the parents of one gravely ill child carried on a conversation at his beside. They discussed at length the gloomy prognosis, unaware that he probably understood most of what they were saying.

Whether through such incidents or in other ways, it is common for seriously ill children to understand the life-threatening nature of their situations. Although there is a natural reluctance to talk to a child about topics such as death or disability, this hesitancy often results from adult taboos on discussing these topics with children, rather than from the young patient's lack of awareness.

Avoiding discussion of troubling topics with a seven-year-old boy doesn't mean the child is not thinking about them, it just means he is being told to keep his thoughts to himself. A hospitalized child is likely to make the worst possible interpretation when others avoid honest discussion. Having to keep dread concerns inside simply adds to the burden of a child who is experiencing a serious medical condition. Even when the outlook is grim, children are likely to feel less afraid if they understand what is happening. It is better for them to have the opportunity to discuss their fears, although such conversations may be troubling to the adults involved.

Hiding your feelings from a child is very difficult. Even if you don't say what is on your mind, children are very perceptive of adult behaviors such as finger drumming, finger chewing, eye watering and sobbing. Research has shown that such nonverbal expressions of parental tension maintain high levels of distress in four- to ten-year-old patients.

Should you find yourself crying or otherwise in obvious distress, explain your feelings to the young patient. You might say something like"I know you aren't feeling good and I am sad because you are having such a rough time." Such a comment explains your emotional reaction and may encourage similar self-disclosure from the child.

Being accepting and nonjudgmental is important when providing emotional support to a young person. For instance, while trying to change a child's distorted views of how the symptoms came about, one still should avoid critical or derogatory remarks.

Being nonjudgmental does not mean a sick child should be able to "get away with murder." Hospitalized children sometimes regress and display immature behavior. Whining and complaining may occur in an attempt to manipulate others. Whether the issue is participating in the medical regimen or completing a school assignment, there may need to be a frank discussion about the consequences of inappropriate behavior. For instance, rudeness and constant bell-ringing may encourage the nursing staff to be slow in responding—the opposite effect of what the child hopes to accomplish by such actions.

Although immature behavior should be discouraged, any limitations on the young person should be necessary and realistic. Unnecessary restrictions simply add to the stress on the child. For example, the mother of one eleven-year-old patient frequently criticized his choice of reading material. He recalled that her visits usually included a lecture on "why I shouldn't read super hero comic books or *Mad Magazine*."

In addition to realistic privileges in areas such as reading material, the young person should be given appropriate freedom in other areas. For instance, the child should be allowed as much activity as is possible, since it often is hard for an energetic youngster to comply with the physical restrictions of the hospital regimen.

Self-care should be encouraged. Although mistakes will be made along the way, it is important to praise the child's positive efforts. Such encouragement is an important way of supporting the young patient's adaptive coping.

To further combat feelings of helplessness, the child should be given as much decision-making control as is possible. For example, if a special activity or treat is to be arranged, it may be appropriate to let the young person select what it will be.

Providing autonomy does not mean pampering. When overindulgence occurs, it sometimes comes more from the needs of the adult than from those of the young patient. For instance, if one blames oneself for the child's condition, the desire to make amends may result in being overly protective or overly lenient.

But guilt about the child's condition also can have the opposite effect. On occasion an adult will deal with self-blame by rejecting the hospitalized child. Such an adult becomes uncooperative and detached from the patient. This kind of rejection may be demonstrated by behaviors such as forgetting medical instructions or blaming complications on the child.

Clearly, sharing guilt feelings with another adult is better than unintentionally letting those emotions result in either overindulgence or neglect of the young patient. If you are experiencing such self-blame and have been keeping it inside, consider sharing your thoughts and emotions with someone; your burden of secrecy will be lifted, and you may discover new ways of coping with the demands you are facing. On the other hand, if you know an adult who appears to be either overindulging or neglecting a child, consider offering to talk with that person. Having someone reach out may be just what that individual needs right now.

Brothers and sisters can be concerned for their sick sibling, while at the same time harbor feelings of resentment. The time and money expended for the hospitalized child may lessen opportunities for the other children. Even when siblings support such sacrifices, there are likely to be feelings of ambivalence; they may willingly give up opportunities but still have a sense of loss or of being cheated. Perceiving such selfishness in oneself can lead to feelings of guilt in the healthy child. But both resentment and guilt tend to be expressed in disguised forms rather than directly. For example, a child may throw a tantrum about not being able to go on a planned outing, without ever expressly blaming the hospitalized sibling as the reason for the cancellation. To lessen the disruption due to such pent up feelings, family members should have opportunities to openly share their concerns and regrets.

In two-parent families, parents can take turns visiting the hospitalized child so that the other family members continue to receive the support they need. One-parent families in such situations can obtain valuable support from close friends and relatives. If you know a single parent who has a hospitalized child, you might consider offering to perform household chores, run errands, or care for siblings of the patient.

During periods of stress, there may be a need to set aside time to be with one another. For example, in addition to sharing meals, family members can go for walks or play games that allow conversation. Such opportunities for one-to-one interaction can help to minimize disruptions due to the hospitalization.

Patients in Intensive Care Units

- Visiting my father in the intensive care unit was "psychologically devastating...to me. [There was] no privacy for patient or visitor. [It was a] frightening experience to the uninitiated visitor."

Conditions are quite different from a general medical floor if your friend or loved one is in an intensive care unit (ICU) or similar special care unit. There may be individual rooms, but many units employ an "amphitheater" format with several beds and few, if any, partitions. There is a mass of medical equipment that may seem to have a life of its own: control lights flash; video monitors blip and beep; respirators whoosh; and suction pumps gurgle.

A variety of wires and tubes attach the machines to the patients whose lives they maintain and monitor. But in contrast to the animated machinery, ICU patients tend to be pale, still and quiet.

Your interactions with the person will be in the presence of staff members who frequently check both the machinery and the attached patient. One of these professionals will be the patient's primary nurse—a good person to check with when you want information about the patient. You will notice that there are more nurses than in a similar space on a general medical floor. You also may find that they wear special clothing—such as green surgical attire—to decrease the possibility of contamination. The object of all this mechanization, specialization and attention are the four or eight or twelve patients, all of whom have life-threatening conditions.

It is not unusual to be disturbed by the strange noises, sights and smells of the ICU. When my wife was a teenager she volunteered as a candy striper in a hospital. As a pharmacy aide, she made deliveries throughout the hospital, but there was one destination where she never lingered—the ICU. Although she made many trips there, she never got over the uneasy feeling she experienced when confronted with it's unique appearance and gravely ill patients.

In addition to the surroundings being disturbing, the behavior of the patient can cause concern. A frequent occurrence is the development of what has come to be called an "ICU psychosis."

Disorientation and confusion are common aspects of the ICU psychosis that many patients develop. When this temporary thought disorder occurs, it is brought on by conditions experienced in the ICU. These stressors include the continuous noise of people and machines, as well as round-the-clock lighting. Restful sleep in such a setting may be difficult or impossible. In addition to the light and noise, the patient's illness and medication can contribute to the disorientation. For instance, any patient with a high fever or under sedation will find it hard to think clearly.

A patient experiencing an ICU psychosis may have hallucinations (false sensory perceptions) or delusions (false beliefs). The person may make sense one moment but not the next. Although an ICU psychosis can be very disturbing to both you and the patient, the condition has two positive aspects: (1) since it is the result of factors experienced in the ICU, it will dissipate in the absence of those stressors; (2) as you will see, there are a number of ways you can help the patient to increase awareness and orientation.

Special Considerations

Visiting a patient in the ICU, despite the surroundings, may be well worth the effort. You can offer something that no staff member can give—a link to the familiar reality of life outside the hospital.

Focus most of your visit on what is happening in the outside world. Your visit to an intensive care unit patient can be a vital contact between the person and the continuing flow of life. There are several things you can do to help establish that link. Mention what day it is and what time it is. Describe the weather. Talk about positive events, such as amusing news stories or happenings involving friends and relatives. Even seemingly mundane events are likely to be interesting to the person. Knowledge of routine occurrences becomes very valuable when one is cut off from the routine.

While working at a Veterans Administration hospital I was asked to see a patient with myasthenia gravis. This disease causes weakening of the muscles but often can be effectively controlled with appropriate medication. Without the medication though, the person becomes extremely weak. The patient I was to see was scheduled for a period in which he would be taken off his medication. Since he had no friends or family to visit him, I was to be his surrogate support system. I met with him a couple of times prior to the medication change and we established a friendly relationship. Then he was taken off his medicine and transferred to the ICU. While he was in the unit I visited him daily. Although he could not write or talk, he acknowledged my presence by squeezing my hand and by giving me slight head nods. I did the talking—mostly about the weather and sports—and he listened. Although they were short and simple, these visits played an important role in his recovery.

There are a number of alternatives to conversation if communication is difficult. You can offer a felt-tipped pen and a pad if the patient understands you but has difficulty talking. (A felt-tipped pen is preferable to a pencil because it requires less pressure, and it is better than a ballpoint pen because it need not be pointing downward for a continuous flow of ink.) When writing is not possible, an alphabet board provides an alternative means of forming words. Although there are alphabet boards with magnetic letters, it may be faster to simply supply a listing of the alphabet and let the patient form words by pointing to the appropriate letters. If the person is conscious but can't spell or talk, keep your queries to one closed question at a time. For example, "Is there anything you want me to tell the staff?" or "Is there anything you want me to find out about?" Arrange for the patient to respond in a way that will be easiest for the person; possibilities include head nods, eye blinks or hand squeezes.

Even if the patient is unresponsive, the staff may encourage you to carry on a one-way conversation—the same idea already discussed with regard to unresponsive children. For example, one woman told me about visiting her sister in an ICU. "We were encouraged [by the staff] to talk to her because they felt she could hear, but not really respond, and that it would help her to come out of her coma—which she eventually did and fully recovered."

Nurse Margaret Ann Chatham conducted some interesting research on improving the support provided to intensive care patients. Her focus was on wives visiting their husbands in the ICU following coronary bypass surgery. She randomly assigned ten patients to an experimental group and ten patients to a control group. The wives of the ten men in the experimental group listened to an audio tape that explained the purpose of the ICU equipment and the nature of the postoperative care. The tape also advised the woman to make eye contact with her husband, to touch him frequently, and to mention the time, who she was and where they were.

The wives received the last set of instructions because post-heart-surgery patients often experience difficulties with memory, judgment and emotional control; such patients also tend to have problems knowing where they are, what time it is, and the identity of those around them. Nurse Chatham believed that these symptoms would be reduced by the wives making eye contact with their husbands, touching them, and orienting them to time, place and person.

During the first four days after surgery, the patients' wives made three 10-minute visits each day. Also three times a day, a nurse rated each patient on a variety of behavioral measures.

Patients in the experimental group received ratings that were significantly more favorable in five categories of behavior. Compared to the control-group patients, these men were: better oriented to time, place and person; more appropriate in their actions; less confused; less likely to experience delusions; and more likely to sleep for longer periods.

If you are visiting an intensive care patient, you may want to offer the same kind of support advocated by nurse Chatham.

☐ Make eye contact with the patient, if the person's eyes are open.
☐ Frequently touch the person. Give a friendly pat or hold the person's hand.
☐ During each visit mention who you are and where you are, as well as the day and time.

A variety of restrictions may apply to visitors. As one ICU visitor told me: "I felt very restricted....There were so many rules—only certain people could visit at a certain time."

Almost all intensive care units have a limit of two visitors at a time. Often, only immediate family members are allowed to visit. Children usually are discouraged from visiting, but most units will allow children to visit in certain situations. Hospitals usually have restrictions on the frequency of visits; the most common limitations being every hour, every two hours or at scheduled times (such as 10 a.m., 2 p.m. and 8 p.m.). The duration of these visits also tends to be limited to brief periods, typically ranging from 5 to 30 minutes.

The more concerned one is about the severity of a patient's condition, the greater the need to visit the person frequently. Consequently, the visiting restrictions of an ICU may seem to be especially harsh. But don't assume that flexibility is impossible. Most hospitals will allow exceptions to visiting restrictions in response to special needs of the patient and family. If you desire greater access to the patient, make your wishes known to a staff member. Probably the best individual to talk with is the ICU charge nurse, since that person usually is the professional responsible for allowing exceptions to the visiting regulations.

In addition to restrictions on the amount of visiting, there are likely to be limitations on what you are allowed to bring into the ICU. For instance, gifts of food and flowers usually are not allowed. These rules are not likely to be broken easily, with the possible exception of the staff allowing some special food for a patient who has begun to eat again.

Being transferred out of an ICU is usually a positive sign that means the person is getting better. Although one may be excited about the improved prognosis, it also is common for both patients and loved ones to feel apprehensive. In the ICU the person has been constantly monitored by sophisticated equipment and has been closely attended to by a specialized staff. Fear of what the future will bring makes sense when one considers the patient is leaving behind much of the staff and equipment responsible for keeping the person alive during the past several days. On the new ward there will be less equipment, and the person will be just one of many patients for whom the staff must provide care.

Visits from a loved one may be vital during this transition period. Appropriate moral and decision-making support can do a great deal to ease the patient's mind, as well as your own.

Psychiatric Patients

- My sister-in-law was hospitalized for depression. "We would discuss family members, things that my family was doing, how [she] was getting along and what she had been doing as an inpatient at the hospital....I was disappointed that [she] was not doing as well as I had hoped for....I would like [her] to realize that she ...could be living a normal life if she would just let her physician help her. I would like to discuss this more with [her] and as always I would offer my help in any way possible."
- I visited my schizophrenic friend 20 times in the hospital. "We discussed what was going on in each of our lives....We talked about the patient's animals and her daughter. We also played ping-pong and looked at an art museum....It brought me closer to [her] and it also helped me understand her illness better by talking to the doctors. We became more aware of each others' needs for getting along."

Removal from the home environment is one of the goals when a person is hospitalized for psychiatric reasons. Since family members and friends represent part of that environment, you may be discouraged from seeing the patient during the early part of the hospitalization. But as the person moves toward increased stability, it is therapeutic to gradually reestablish contact with friends and family. Since it is difficult for you to know the extent of the patient's recovery, take your lead from the staff. For instance, you can call the nurses' station and ask about the advisability of a visit. If the person is not yet ready for visitors, you can ask if there is some other way in which you could help the patient. You might be able to bring something from the person's home or there may be a gift that you can leave for the patient.

Once the staff members approve a visit from you, continue to look to them for guidance. Ask how you can best contribute to the patient's recovery.

Make your first visits short. Renewing your relationship in small doses may be the best approach for both of you, especially if the person you encounter seems quite different from the one you have known.

Some of the patient's behavior may seem confusing and illogical, making contact difficult. Realize that the person is in the midst of recovery, and that the staff members believe it now is appropriate for you to begin to renew your relationship. That renewal is likely to have its ups and downs, but now is the time to start your rebuilding efforts.

Brain Injury and Stroke Patients

- My friend was injured in a car accident and "almost died. I showed him some pictures I had with me and I told him of some of the activities I was currently involved with. He told me about the accident and the therapy he was currently receiving."
- After a massive stroke, my grandmother had a "brain operation. She was disoriented and the family tried to help her remember her past."

- My brother was in a motorcycle accident. I visited three times but "he was not too receptive, and sometimes he even became hostile. I did not understand why he acted this way."

Damage to the brain is one common reason for hospitalization. Two frequently occurring kinds of damage are stroke (also called cerebrovascular accident or CVA) and traumatic brain injury.

A stroke means that part of the brain's blood supply has been cut off. When that happens, body regions fail to function if they are controlled by the affected area of the brain.

Traumatic brain injury results from a blow to the head or from lack of oxygen. As with a stroke, there will be a loss of function in those areas controlled by the damaged region.

In addition to the loss of physical abilities, there also may be changes in the person's usual ways of thinking and feeling. For instance, the verbal abilities of a patient may be affected so that the person uses incorrect words or has difficulty understanding words spoken by others.

As you can imagine, the loss of such abilities can be very disheartening. Patients may become frustrated, irritable and angry. But reacting to the loss of function is not the only way emotions can be affected. The brain damage itself can cause changes in the person's emotional makeup. Such direct effects can be extremely varied—ranging from depression to inappropriate elation and from apathy to stubbornness.

The patient you visit may seem very different from the individual you knew prior to the hospitalization. In fact, research consistently shows that the most troubling problem to the close relatives of traumatic brain injury patients is the personality change in their loved ones.

Remember that the person may have difficulty thinking and that such patients have a double risk of emotional disturbance—both as a reaction to the loss of function and as a direct consequence of the brain damage. Since the person's behavior may be disconcerting at times, here are some ideas to keep in mind when visiting a brain injury or stroke victim.

- ☐ Try to be patient. The person probably is striving hard to overcome the loss of function.
- ☐ Talk slowly and distinctly, but don't shout. Try writing notes if spoken words don't seem to make sense to the person.
- ☐ Use closed questions if communication is difficult. Be sure to avoid multiple questions. (See Chapter 3.)
- ☐ Bring reminders of home and of life on the outside. For instance, photos of current happenings at familiar places can be helpful.

Terminal Patients

- "In my last visit with my aunt I had the opportunity to speak to her for about five minutes before she got tired again, and I used this time to tell her I loved her. I felt so relieved to be able to have done that, especially since her situation was terminal. The funeral was still a very gloomy day, but the simple fact that aunt ____ knew we all loved her made it easier."
- "I have been visiting my sister's husband who two weeks ago was diagnosed as having cancer...that has already spread [throughout his body]....These are difficult visits [but I believe they] show the person I care....[My husband's] father died of cancer when he was 52 (my brother-in-law is 54) and [my husband] remembers being very hurt when several good friends of his parents 'just couldn't' go to see his father in the hospital before he died."
- "This feeling [of death] makes it very difficult for me to visit people in the hospital. I feel that this might be the last time I see

them if they are seriously ill. The thought of death terrifies me. I don't like facing death."

What are we facing when we confront death? There are many different opinions.

I recently led a workshop on suicide prevention for staff members of Pennsylvania juvenile detention centers. We held the sessions in the large conference room of a motel. The topic for the second day of the meeting was intervening with suicidal individuals. During a discussion concerning the consequences of suicide, we began talking about the finality of death. After considering various religious beliefs concerning life after death, I brought up the viewpoint that existence ends at death. To demonstrate this idea, I asked one of the participants to switch off the room lights. Since the facility also served as a disco, he had some difficulty locating the correct controls among the various switches for the lighting system. While he continued to search, I presented the analogy that some believe death is like turning off the lights—it is a quiet, peaceful nonexistence.

Just as I finished describing the analogy the lights dimmed, but the participants gasped as the room suddenly filled with sparkling light from a brilliant mirrored ball in the ceiling. At that point we all wondered whether the discussion had been joined by the preeminent Advocate for the heavenly viewpoint.

No one knows for a fact what death is like. But most views on what happens after death can be classified into four major categories.

- ☐ Death is quiet, peaceful nonexistence. This is the belief I was demonstrating when interrupted by the sparkling light.
- ☐ The essence of the personality survives in the form of an immortal soul.

- [ ] At some point in the future the body will be reconstituted and restored to life.
- [ ] An aspect of the personality will be reincarnated in another life form and live again on earth.

The latter three views all involve religious faith. But faith means there is no factual way of demonstrating the belief. In the absence of concrete evidence, even the most religious person can have doubts about exactly what death will bring.

Burdensome thoughts sometimes are expressed directly by a terminal patient. In other cases the person may approach troubling topics more indirectly. For instance, a child may ask "What would happen if a plane crashed into my room?" or "What happens to a dog when it is run over by a car?" The best kind of response to such a question is reflection. You can clarify what really is being asked with a statement such as "You want to know what happens when we die." Making that kind of reflection takes courage, but being willing to frankly confront the topic can help the patient share a tremendous burden.

Death can be seen as the release from suffering or one can choose to "risk death" by agreeing to a dangerous medical procedure. But no one looks forward to death.

Even when life is full of pain and suffering, we know what it means to live. But death is different; it is the unknown. Although death is just as much a part of life as birth, its unknown aspect makes death harder to accept.

The burden of facing the unknown can be lightened by the presence of friends and loved ones. Regardless of what one believes about death, it is reassuring to know that one's life has made a difference. It can be comforting to see that contributions one has made will continue to affect those whose lives continue.

Special Considerations

Learning that the patient's condition is terminal is stressful for the hospitalized person, friends and family. Common feelings at the time of the diagnosis include shock, disbelief, anger, fear and despair. Being unable to ward off death, there can be a sense of futility or helplessness. There may be dreams and goals for which there now is no hope of ever attaining. Vital relationships are going to end.

When there is gradual deterioration, the patient may become tired of the condition, tired of being hospitalized, and tired of the pain and discomfort. Likewise, you may grow weary of lengthy or repeated hospitalizations, weary of seeing the patient in pain, or weary of the pressure placed on your family. Even if both you and the patient wish for an end, you may feel guilty about wanting the patient to die. In such situations you may feel you should be stronger, kinder, or more generous. But despite a desire to be superhuman, you may find that you too are merely mortal.

When the patient's medical condition slowly worsens, self-worth is threatened as the person loses physical abilities and role responsibilities, all the while becoming more dependent upon others. As dependency increases, so may anxiety over a host of questions. What will death be like? Will I face it alone? How bad will my physical condition become before I die? How much pain will there be? For instance, one woman discussed a variety of topics with her dying sister: "When is pain too much? When is permanent sleep better than fighting? Her fear. The difference between letting go and holding on."

When a patient anticipates the end of life as we know it, there is mourning over the loss of relationships and the things of this world. Such mourning may include guilt over the hurt and difficulty one's death will cause those who are close.

Some patients become so overwhelmed by self-doubt,

anxiety or grief that they withdraw into themselves in unreachable isolation. Others strive to cope by denying the reality of their situation. Eventually, many patients come to terms with these issues and are able to face death with either a sense of resignation or an attitude of acceptance.

Coping with self-doubt, anxiety and grief is much easier if there are supportive family and friends who allow the patient to openly share concerns, while at the same time expressing their own affection and regard for the person. Withdrawal and isolation become more likely if such support is not available, as in cases where the terminal prognosis has been "withheld" from the patient.

Who should know of a terminal diagnosis? There are a variety of opinions. Some believe such a diagnosis should be withheld from the dying patient to avoid "unnecessary" grief. Others believe that as soon as the prognosis is medically certain, the patient has a right to know that death is expected; having possession of such knowledge allows one to prepare in the best ways possible. Similar arguments exist with regard to telling the patient's dependent children, other relatives, and friends. In each case, those in possession of the bad news will have to make their own decisions regarding whom to tell.

But such information is hard to keep secret. One man described being told "by my son's surgeon that the biopsy proved he had inoperable cancer, and that I was not to tell him....YOU CANNOT HIDE SUCH A DIAGNOSIS for even one hour after the patient has recovered from the anesthesia."

Others—including an "uninformed" patient—often deduce the reality of the situation. Although they still may pretend as though they do not know the prognosis, since those who have the information apparently do not want to discuss it.

Keeping a terminal diagnosis under wraps has much more to do with the needs of those possessing the knowledge than with protecting those who do not know. After the prognosis becomes known or the person dies, those who have been kept in the dark are likely to feel betrayed by those who have withheld the information.

The terminal patient may want to affirm contact with you. This may include seeking assurance that you understand, making eye contact, and touching or holding you. Clinging to you is one way the person can cope with the thought of death and the loss of your relationship. Sometimes the need to touch comes from fear of being abandoned. Whatever its source, it is a normal reaction to such tragic circumstances.

You too may need to cling to the person who is facing death. As with the patient, such a desire is normal for loved ones.

When possible, it can be helpful to share the feelings that are behind the need to make contact with one another. It takes courage on your part to engage in such honest talk, but open and frank sharing can move the interaction toward enhanced understanding.

Honest communication can initiate problem solving regarding those circumstances that can be modified. Even when a patient's survival or recovery clearly are impossible, setting limited goals that are within reach provides a realistic sense of hope. Working on such tasks can aid coping in a number of ways: attention is focused on concrete realities and away from anxieties; there are interactions with others and with the environment that demonstrate the person still is a part of this world; reaching the goals often gives a sense of mastery and control that enhances dignity and self-esteem. Being productive, even in limited ways, may give a feeling of achievement that helps to ease the loss of traditional work and family roles.

You may be able to aid the patient with some tasks—without usurping the person's responsibilities or those of the staff. You also may want to seek information about the likely course of the patient's condition. Participating in the person's care and gathering information about what is to come can help you to feel useful and more in control. For instance, when one woman visited her dying mother, they sometimes talked about "things she wanted to be done or wanted me to do, both in the present and after her death."

There may come a time when there is little you can do for the person. But there might be other individuals who could benefit from your caring and support. Productive contributions on your part may include listening to their concerns and aiding them with problem solving. You may find that such interactions can end up helping you as much as the other person. Providing concrete assistance to others enables you to make a contribution even though the patient may be beyond your help. Doing something for others can give a sense of being productive in a situation where you may have begun to feel helpless.

It is adaptive to maintain hope. But rather than hope for recovery, it now may be hope for the patient to be comfortable and hope for the well-being of those who are close. You can maintain such hope by continuing to make your short-term contributions, while moving toward acceptance of the inevitable loss you are about to face.

Helping the patient and others with their immediate needs allows you to cope with the situation one day at a time, but you still may need to start planning for what the future will bring. And so will the patient. While you continue to cherish the person, the patient may need your permission to begin separating from you. And as you continue expressing affection, you also may need to begin allowing yourself to gradually detach from the individual.

Even as you continue meeting your daily responsibilities, you should have an outlet for sharing your grief and other feelings. While you may have encouraged other loved ones to share with you, there may come a time when you need such support yourself. With a caring person, you may need to search for the meaning or purpose of the patient's impending death. You also may have unpleasant feelings to share, such as fear, helplessness, anger or guilt.

Some of the negative feelings you express may relate to the staff. When appropriate, you should act on your feelings. But at the same time, you must remember that the staff members are only human and that their technology has its limitations.

Participating in the choice to end medical treatment for a terminal patient is the ultimate in decision-making support. It also may be one of the most difficult kinds of support to provide.

Medical technology has changed the definition of death. At one time a person was considered dead when there was no heartbeat or respiration, but now machines often can maintain these functions. Consequently, the medical profession has developed the concept of brain death. Key elements in brain death are:

- a deep coma causing the person to be unresponsive;
- no independent respiration or spontaneous reflexes for 6 to 12 hours;

and
- the reason for the coma is known and is judged to be irreversible.

A number of burdensome questions may arise when a patient is close to death. For example: When does one conclude that the condition is irreversible? How do you incorporate the patient's wishes into the medical plan? What are the financial costs resulting from continuation of "heroic measures" such as respirators and cardiac resuscitation?

Crucial questions like these are best discussed with a person who is coherent and possesses sound judgment. As a rational individual, I may specify conditions under which I would want an end to medical efforts on my behalf. A formalized example of this is a "living will" in which I can express those desires in writing. Such a document is legally binding in some states but not in others.

A document that is binding in most states is a durable power of attorney. (It is called "durable" because it continues to be valid even if the person who granted it becomes incompetent.) If I am competent, I can delegate the authority to make all medical decisions that I could make for myself, including decisions that may permit me to die of natural causes.

But some individuals are reluctant to grant such sweeping power. If I am hesitant to delegate such broad decision-making responsibility, I can be more specific in the authority that I assign to another. For instance, I can specify that the person with my power of attorney can make decisions regarding whether I should have surgery requiring general anesthesia, whether I should have a limb amputated, or whether various specified extraordinary means should be used to maintain my life.

A durable power of attorney (in most states) or a living will (in some states) serves to clarify and define the decision-making process during a very difficult time. But whether or not the person wants a legally binding document, the dying patient may wish to discuss issues associated with the termination of medical treatment. Although entering into such a discussion requires courage, it may be important to give the individual an opportunity to express desires concerning the extent of life-prolonging medical efforts.

When effective communication with the patient is not possible, input from other sources will have to suffice. The attending physician and close family members are likely to be the most important contributors when a decision must be made without the patient's participation.

When a Patient Dies

- "My father was the strongest man I ever saw....Even though he was in pain he always had a very pretty smile on his face. Everyone who knew him remembered that smile."

Death means the patient's struggle is over, but life goes on for the survivors. You and others close to the person will need time to mourn the loss. Although painful, it will be helpful to openly express your feelings to someone who will listen and understand.

It is normal to experience any of a wide range of reactions in response to the death of a person close to you. You may spend time in sad reminiscing. Sometimes there will be regret over lost opportunities; you may feel either guilt or anger over these, depending upon whom you believe to be at fault. If your anger is directed toward the deceased person, you may be ashamed of having a feeling that seems inappropriate. On the other hand, as you discuss the qualities of the deceased, you may find yourself idealizing aspects of your relationship. Feeling the full impact of the death may result in despair about the loss or lead to anxiety regarding other deaths to come—including your own and those of other loved ones. When you are confronted with such tragic issues, usual daily activities may seem meaningless or worthless; you may experience resentment toward others who appear to be living happily. Again, none of these reactions are either strange or abnormal.

Depending upon the role the deceased person played in your life, you may feel bewildered or adrift. For example, if you usually counted on the person for help in making decisions, there now is a need to reallocate decision-making responsibilities. Such a reordering in no way diminishes the significance of the deceased person's contributions to your life, but the realignment does enable you to handle new choices to be made.

Trying out new patterns of behavior can produce fears and anxieties. For a time the consequences of your efforts may be in doubt, and there is likely to be a good deal of trial and error. Be willing to reach out for the support you need in order to cope with the continuing demands of life.

Adjusting to life without the deceased individual may be a slow process. During the first year, special dates such as birthdays, anniversaries and holidays may bring a renewed sense of loss. Experiencing these times without the person may not seem quite right. It is appropriate on such occasions to reminisce about how things used to be. Being sad or tearful is a common occurrence.

Memories you cherish from your interactions will continue to be a part of you. Those recollections will not be changed by confronting new demands or by developing new relationships.

In time the pain subsides and it becomes easier to recall the person without also feeling the grief of the loss. When that begins to happen, you will be on the way to an adaptive resolution of your bereavement.

Confronting death may tax the coping skills of patient and visitor alike, and there are numerous other patient-related developments that can be overwhelming. The next chapter discusses such crises and how to deal with them.

7

Dealing With Hospital Crises

- The most negative aspect of my hospital stay was the "pain [and] discomfort."
- The worst part of my hospitalization was "being away from my home and family."
- "Completely depending on…someone for help is a terrible feeling."
- The most difficult part of being in the hospital was "the time spent just waiting."
- "Depending on what the patient's ailment is, it can have a real sobering and depressing effect. It can be a very stressful situation" for the visitor.
- It was difficult "to realize that the patient was getting no better."
- I am bothered by "the anxiety of wondering how the hospitalization will go and [by] frustration of knowing there is not much you can do to help. You are especially upset when visiting a family member."
- I found it hard when "my uncle was so sick he did not recognize me the entire time I was there."
- "I hated seeing my grandmother hooked up to those machines."

This chapter focuses on circumstances that have the potential to overstress you or the patient. A crisis is a period of change during which one's usual ways of coping are not sufficient to alleviate the difficulties. It is a turning point in one's life that brings overwhelming demands.

Hospitalization as a Crisis for the Patient

The stresses accompanying a hospital stay can overtax the patient's coping skills. Common pressures include: experiencing distressing symptoms and procedures, separation from one's usual lifestyle, loss of control, and confronting the unknown.

Distressing Symptoms and Procedures

- "The most negative aspect [of being in the hospital] was the pain experienced."
- "Mostly, I didn't like the pain and discomfort."
- The worst part of being hospitalized was "the pain of the tests I went through."
- "There were many unpleasant and painful tests."
- "I couldn't eat for a couple of days and also I was in pain."
- The most negative aspects of my hospital stay were "the operation itself, shots, IV's and being away from home."
- The "pain [and] nausea [were the worst part of my hospitalization]. I couldn't get warm post-op."
- "The IV site was in my right hand this last time, and, as I am a right-handed person, I was greatly limited."
- The worst part of being in the hospital was "that I didn't have my sight."
- The most negative aspect of my hospitalization was "feeling weak and having nothing work to make me stronger, except time."

Pain, nausea, disfigurement and loss of abilities are intrinsically disturbing experiences often associated with hospitalizations. Also, the extent of one's weakness due to illness or surgery can cause dismay, especially if the person was in relatively good health shortly before the hospitalization.

Separation

- "I didn't have very many visitors."
- The most unpleasant aspect of my hospital stay was "being away from home."
- The most negative aspect of my hospitalization stay was "being away from family."
- The worst part of being in the hospital was "that I was away from my children and couldn't see them."
- I was "anxious to go home."
- The worst aspect of being hospitalized was "missing school and work—also the pain."
- I don't like the "long times you have to spend alone."
- "It got pretty lonely at times. It wasn't like home."

It is easy for a hospitalized individual to feel disconnected from events that continue without the person's usual participation. Separation from one's normal roles can result in feelings of alienation or isolation.

Loss of Control

- The worst aspect of my hospitalization was "being immobile in the cast and having to rely on others for everything."
- I didn't like the "feelings of vulnerability/dependence [or the] loss of mobility/freedom."
- The most negative apects of my hospital stay were "coping with the pain [and the] lack of privacy."
- I disliked being "confined to bed [and having a] liquid diet for three days."

- The worst part of being in the hospital was "the lack of sleep due to medicine administered throughout the day and night."
- "Everyone kept waking me up and not letting me alone!"

Being ill or injured robs much of the control to which the person has been accustomed. It can be shocking to suddenly find oneself at the mercy of a disease or disability. Even more autonomy is lost when one is hospitalized. Whatever degree of control the individual had outside the hospital is decreased by becoming an inpatient; the person now receives numerous directives concerning what to do and what not to do.

And while one is inside the hospital, life on the outside continues. Not only does a patient lose much of the control over the immediate envrionment, but outside of the hospital others may begin moving into the person's traditional roles. Any of these loses can be a blow to one's sense of autonomy and self-esteem.

The Unknown

- "I was sick and didn't know how things were going to come out."
- The worst part of being hospitalized was my "initial concern/apprehension/fear."
- The most negative aspect of being in the hospital was "...the fear and anguish [associated with] discovering I had cancer."
- The worst parts of my hospitalization were "waiting to be scheduled for tests [and] waiting for test results."
- The most negative aspect of my hospital stay was "not understanding everything that was being done."
- I "had to be sent to another hospital to find" out the reason for some of my health problems.
- "The cost of hospital care is very expensive."

A host of uncertainties may be associated with the patient's hospitalization. Will I live or die? What is causing my symptoms? What will the staff be doing to me? Why will they be doing it? What will be the results? How much pain will there be and how long will it last? Will I lose abilities I've counted on? Will I get better? How long will I be here? What will recuperation be like? Will there be a recurrence of the problem? What will happen to those who usually depend upon me? Will I be a burden on others? How will I look? How much will this cost and how will I pay for it?

Any of these stresses can be sufficient to overtax the coping skills of a hospitalized individual. But patients may not be the only ones under pressure.

Hospitalization as a Crisis for Visitors

In addition to being a stressful experience for the patient, a hospitalization can be a crisis situation for friends and family members. We frequently worry more about others than we do about ourselves. For instance, research shows that mothers usually are more concerned about their children's health than their own.

Close friends and family members frequently have difficulty adapting to the patient's hospitalization and often experience unpleasant emotions. Such distressing feelings may include anxiety, fear, despair, anger or helplessness.

The pressures that can lead to a crisis depend upon the nature and duration of the hospitalization. Common stresses include: the initial shock, uncertainty about the future, hospital restrictions, problems arising from supporting a distressed patient, the patient's appearance and behavior, and difficulties associated with serious illness.

Shock

- "In the beginning when they are very sick, it can be depressing."
- It is difficult "seeing my brother-in-law so impatient to be up and about and knowing that only a miracle will allow that to happen."
- The most negative aspect of visiting the hospital was "learning how serious my uncle's operation really was."
- The worst part of going to the hospital was "when I visited my dad and he couldn't talk to me or hold me. It was depressing to see that man so weak and sick."

If the friend or loved one has been in good health, hospitalization will come as a shock. It may seem incomprehensible that a person who was well yesterday is now hospitalized. Even when a patient's hospitalization was planned, there still may be shock once a diagnosis is made or when grave developments occur. If the condition is serious, you—as well as the patient—may react with disbelief.

Being in a state of shock makes it difficult or impossible to attend to or remember conversations—especially if they relate to the patient's condition. If others persist in trying to confront us with the critical nature of the situation, we may become angry at them for conveying bad news that we do not want to hear. In most cases, such overwhelming shock and denial subside within a day. But if the patient's condition remains serious and worrying is compounded by lack of sleep, then one may continue in a state of shock for several days.

Uncertainty

Here are the responses several visitors gave when asked to describe the most negative aspect of visiting someone in the hospital.

- "The fear of their condition worsening and actually seeing them

sick."
- "Apprehension of the unknown concerning the condition of the patient."
- "Knowing that they are in pain and fearing setbacks."
- "...waiting for results of tests."
- "Not knowing if there was something seriously wrong."

Immediate reactions in the early stages of the hospitalization include fear that the person will die or relief that the patient is not worse off. Hope for a good recovery may be accompanied by dread that the person's condition will worsen. Even after recovery is underway, there may be fear that the condition will recur.

If the patient's condition becomes stabilized and recovery seems likely, it is natural to wonder about residual effects. How long will this hospitalization last? Will future hospitalizations be necessary? Will there be continuing disabilities?

Often there is a need to understand a reason for the person's condition. What caused it? How could it have been prevented?

One may feel responsible in some way for the person's plight; there may be a need to review the events leading to the hospitalization and consider whether one should have done something differently. Were there early symptoms that were missed? Were there interventions that should have been tried? We sometimes blame ourselves for not having prevented the situation that led to the person being in the hospital. In addition to events prior to the hospitalization, there also is a tendency to examine efforts since the admission and to wonder whether we should have acted differently in some way.

Restrictions

- "I feel the visiting hours are not long enough for certain types of patients."

- "The hours are often limited and it is difficult to fit it in at times."
- "We were only permitted two to a patient at the one hospital. There were six of us there" so we couldn't all go at once.
- I didn't like "to keep having to get passes as you entered and exited the room. It seemed like you spent more time checking in and out than you did with the patient."

If your contact with the person is limited, you may feel isolated from the patient. The restrictions on your interactions in the hospital may seem quite harsh.

Even the building itself can contribute to a sense of separation. The strangeness and complexity of the hospital may seem overwhelming. Not knowing your way around can be disconcerting whether you are in a small community facility or in a large teaching hospital.

Supporting a Distressed Patient

- "In some cases (when my mom was really sick) it was hard for me to see her in such a bad condition. It really hurt to see her hurting and in such pain."
- It is hard "thinking about or hearing about what has happened or is happening to people. Then how you continue to think about more and more 'bad' things that can happen to someone or yourself."
- "...I felt bad because I couldn't take seeing my sister in pain."
- I felt troubled "listening to someone's hardships and sufferings."

Knowing that a loved one is suffering is stressful. But it can be especially distressing to hear a patient share negative feelings about symptoms, the hospital experience or the future.

The Patient's Appearance and Behavior

Several persons gave the following replies when asked to describe the worst part of visiting someone in the hospital.

- "The most negative aspect [of visiting] was seeing someone I cared for hooked up on tubes."
- "Seeing the person with a lot of tubes going into her body."
- "Seeing someone I love in a great deal of pain and seeing the dramatic loss of weight."
- "When the person is really depressed."
- "Sometimes they are very down on themselves, such as my friend who broke his leg."
- "It was when I visited my grandfather and he could not speak coherently."

The patient's appearance may change dramatically during the hospitalization. Such alterations can be disconcerting, especially if you are not fully prepared for them. For instance, following my throat surgery, my wife was shocked at my gaunt and haggard appearance.

In addition to looking differently, patients sometimes behave in ways that are uncharacteristic for them. For example, one patient in grave condition became delirious. In his confusion he thought it was a time at the beginning of his marriage when he had discovered his wife in an extramarital affair. In fact, the affair had long since ended and the couple's marital difficulties had been resolved years earlier. But during her visits the patient angrily confronted his wife about her infidelity as if it were happening in the present. Needless to say, she was very disturbed by her husband's accusations.

Once he had recovered his faculties, he denied having any suspicions about his wife's fidelity. His angry assertions had resulted from his delirium rather than from any rational analysis. Although a visitor may know that the false beliefs of a delusional patient are not true, it still can be disconcerting to witness such behavior.

Dealing With Hospital Crises

Serious Illness

For several visitors the following experiences were the most negative aspects of seeing someone in the hospital.

- "...having higher expectations of recovery and then finding out the patient has not progressed as much as you had hoped."
- "The feeling of helplessness when you visit someone you love and they are in a lethargic state. You don't know if they can hear or see you."
- "When they are too sick to even know if you're there or not."
- "If they're feeling bad or sick [and] they don't respond."
- "The feeling of helplessness and sadness when someone you love is critically ill."
- "Seeing someone you know as very active in a very helpless state and being unable to do anything about it."
- "The most negative aspect of visiting my dad was that when he was in a lot of pain after surgery I couldn't relieve any of that physical pain. Therefore, I got upset because I felt helpless."

A patient's behavior need not be psychotic in order for it to be very disturbing to you. For example, it can be demoralizing if the person fails to improve, despite the best efforts on everyone's part. Such a lack of progress can lead one to feel powerless and helpless. Or you may feel disheartened if the patient demonstrates no appreciation for your efforts—a circumstance that is especially likely with seriously ill patients.

When a patient is in a coma or heavily sedated, two-way communication is impossible. If the person cannot acknowledge your presence or provide any feedback to you, it is natural to feel frustrated and helpless. Although you might very much want to make things better for the individual, it may seem as though there is nothing meaningful you can do.

Another change sometimes displayed by seriously ill patients is for them to become dependent and demanding.

Having known the person as a self-sufficient individual, it can be confusing to encounter such a transformation. While one wants to help such patients, it is easy to become angry in response to their complaints and apparent ingratitude. When confronted with a demanding or uncooperative person, it is natural to want to leave the room as soon as you have done your duty.

But becoming angry at a hospitalized person somehow seems inappropriate. Catching oneself experiencing such hostile feelings easily can lead to guilt—the shame of resenting a person in medical difficulty who needs your support. Becoming angry at a demanding patient does not mean you are a bad or uncaring person, but it does mean you are human.

The disruptions and changes necessitated by a hospitalization can lead to mental and physical exhaustion. At times, simply getting to the hospital may be a chore, and difficulties associated with transportation can be draining. Even if getting to the hospital is not a problem, the time spent there may necessitate a reordering of priorities at home and a rearrangement of role responsibilities. For example, who will take care of household maintenance tasks such as cleaning, shopping, cooking and taking care of the children. There can be a moratorium with regard to some responsibilities, such as cleaning, but areas such as child care may require a new delegation of responsibilities.

Once a patient appears to be out of danger, you may turn your attention to what recovery will bring. If the patient will have continuing disabilities, there may be concern over the sacrifices required for the sake of the person's rehabilitation. Such sacrifices may involve finances and role responsibilities within the family. Questions may arise such as: How will the bills be paid? Who is going to be the breadwinner? How will child care be handled?

As you can see, a hospitalization is a potential crisis for both patients and visitors. Once a person is in a crisis, some coping efforts are more effective than others.

Patient Coping

Examples of adaptive patient coping include accepting the realities of the situation and seeking information about what to expect. As one looks for ways of dealing with the future, sometimes it is helpful to recall previous crises that have been resolved successfully. Remembering past successes can enhance one's confidence in dealing with the present situation. Another way of gaining strength for the effort ahead is reaching out to family and friends for comfort and assistance.

Patients report that visitors can be important sources of support during times of crisis. Several patients gave the following responses when asked to describe the most positive aspect of having visitors.

- "Having someone you know to talk to."
- "Relieved depression."
- "Tension and stress release."

By providing moral and decision-making support, you can help the patient deal adaptively with the pressures of hospitalization. Controlled studies demonstrate that patients cope much better when they receive such assistance.

Visitor Coping

- "Sometimes if I am upset or uneasy, my feelings are obvious and

therefore make the patient feel uneasy."
- "Sometimes I get really choked up, and I hate having them see that I'm uspet—they're having a hard enough time."
- "After leaving...I felt bad. Also I could see the strain of worry on the other visitors."
- "The most negative aspect [of visiting] would be when my mother was in the hospital. After the first visit, I was so upset over her condition that I could not bring myself up to going back in the course of the next two weeks. I felt so guilty and thought that she would think I didn't care."

A visitor in crisis can communicate emotional turmoil to the patient—whether intended or not. Such a visitor becomes an added strain on the patient and may impede recovery.

It is common for visitors to feel ambivalent toward patients. You may be discouraged but want to convey encouragement; you may feel doubtful but want to communicate confidence. But patients receiving baseless encouragement and illogical confidence quickly perceive the true discomfort felt by friends and family.

Many visitors believe the best ways to help a patient are to be constantly cheerful, to avoid any in-depth discussion of the person's condition, to tell the individual everything will be all right, and to give advice. But you know that those usually are not helpful responses.

The hospital experience often involves negative thoughts and feelings. For example, it can be scary to think about the risks facing a patient, and one may feel helpless when visiting a patient who is suffering. Attempting to hide fear, feelings of helplessness or other negative emotions makes one very uncomfortable, and such discomfort usually is communicated to patients in unintended ways. Consequently, the cover-up approach takes its toll on both visitors and patients.

Fortunately, there are other ways of handling one's own

distressing feelings. For instance, you can consider sharing negative feelings with the patient. If you are freightened, the patient may prefer to hear an honest admission of your fear rather than being puzzled by your unsuccessful efforts to hide it. Should you feel helpless, it can be appropriate to make a statement like "I feel so frustrated because I can't take away your pain."

When you are having negative reactions, look into yourself and try to identify what you are feeling. Often the honest expression of those unpleasant responses will be much less troubling to the patient than your efforts to cover them over.

Although openly expressing negative thoughts to a patient often is appropriate, there are some reactions that are best not shared with the person. For instance, expressing anger at a patient for being sick may do nothing but hurt the individual. When your common sense tells you that it is best not to confront a patient with certain feelings, you should consider sharing your reactions with someone else.

During a crisis one needs to be able to confide in an accepting person who can be trusted—an individual who will listen to concerns and express understanding. Such a person can help one explore thoughts and feelings, consider options and develop plans.

If you know a visitor who is feeling overwhelmed, it may be appropriate for you to offer the same kinds of moral and decision-making support you have offered the patient. If you are a visitor in crisis, you should seek out such support. But where do you find it? Where do you find a caring, trustworthy, empathic person who will help with problem solving?

As just implied, you may have a friend or relative who can provide appropriate help. In addition to personal acquaintances, there also are human service providers who offer such support. Within the hospital, there may be a social service department that works with the families and friends of patients; in addition to their own staff, these departments often have contact with support groups that may be of help.

Within your community there are likely to be a variety of other helping resources. These probably include crisis intervention and mental health agencies, as well as professionals such as clergy, psychologists and counselors.

Who a person in crisis talks with is not so important as what the would-be helper does. A positive outcome is likely if the intervenor provides empathic, nonjudgmental and honest problem-solving assistance. Such help includes exploring the situation, recognizing emotions, considering alternatives and developing plans. Help from a problem-solving consultant encourages a realistic sense of hope by breaking down difficulties into manageable segments. As progress is made in reaching concrete goals, one begins to have a renewed sense of self-confidence. Feelings of being overwhelmed subside and are replaced with the expectation that one will be able to handle the situation.

This book is intended to be a guide to help you handle many of the stresses associated with being a hospital visitor. But if you need additional assistance you should be willing to seek it out.

In my work as a psychologist, I see many individuals who are feeling overwhelmed by pressures confronting them. In addition to helping such clients productively handle their responsibilities—much like the techniques in this book are intended to help you—I also assist them in developing greater internal control. Two of the self-contol approaches I frequently use are stress inoculation training and relaxation training.

Psychologist Donald Meichenbaum has devised a set of techniques for dealing with anticipated stress. He named the approach "stress inoculation training" because—like an inoculation—you gain a protective benefit by experiencing a little bit of the stress ahead of time.

Meichenbaum says that you can think of any stressful situation as having four phases.

- ☐ **Warning**   I think something bad is going to happen.
- ☐ **Impact**   I was right; I'm in it now.
- ☐ **Arousal**   The stress continues and I begin to worry that I might lose control; I might be overwhelmed.
- ☐ **Reflection**   For now the stress is over, and I am thinking back on how I handled the situation.

You can use Meichenbaum's four phases to categorize the thoughts that you normally have during the stressful episode. First write down the typical self-statements you have during the warning, impact, arousal and reflection stages. Second, make a new list that also is categorized according to the four phases. Include two kinds of entries in the second list.

- ☐ Transfer any statement from the first list that you believe is likely to reduce your stress.
- ☐ Think of other statements you can say to yourself that probably will reduce your stress and add those to the second list as well.

When generating new self-statements for the second list, it is important to record only those thoughts that you truly believe. Avoid propaganda. The tendency to adopt unrealistic self-statements for the second list is the major problem I have encountered when I have helped individuals to use this stress inoculation training technique. Only record a statement in the second list if it really seems plausible to you.

Here are some visitor self-statements that could be replaced by stress-reducing thoughts.

- It bothers me "seeing the equipment, IV's, etc. because I am not used to seeing people dependent...on these instruments."
- "Hospitals are very depressing, seeing others in pain and suffering."

The following example shows how such stressful self-statements can be replaced by stress-reducing thoughts. Using the stress inoculation training approach, I helped this person reduce her distress associated with hospital visits. Prior to trying the technique, she said "I feel apprehensive [while visiting hospitalized patients] since the atmosphere usually makes me feel faint. When I was young and was visiting a sick relative in the hospital, I passed out. Since then I often feel light-headed in hospitals."

During a recent visit to her hospitalized aunt, she ended up shutting herself in the bathroom after she began to cry uncontrollably. Since that experience had been quite distressing, she used the situation of visiting her aunt in implementing the stress inoculation training.

Stress Inoculation Training

First Set	**Second Set**

Warning

How is she? What will she look like?	I know she will not look the way she usually does. I can accept that.
What am I going to talk about? I don't want to say the wrong thing.	I can go over the visit in my mind. I can think about what I'm going to say. I can plan topics of conversation.

Impact

I feel dread as I arrive at the hospital. I feel out of place.	I can take two deep breaths before I get out of the car. Visitors can help patients recover. I am not out of place—I should be here.
I feel like I am in a maze, following a line.	Hospitals are orderly and complex. I can accept that's the way it will be.

Arousal

I don't feel comfortable. I am feeling like I might break down again.	This visit can be different. I can concentrate on the conversation and on tasks like reading her cards and notes.
I feel so self-conscious.	Focusing my attention outwardly on activities helps me stay in control.

Reflection

I wish I had handled things better.	I can learn from this experience and plan for next time.
How will things turn out for her?	Whatever happens, she knows I care and she knows I am thinking of her.

After completing the technique the woman said "I feel very good about the training that we did. I think that visitation is very important. Since I visit people in the hospital in order to make them feel better, I think that it is essential that I don't increase their anxiety....This training will help me handle [my] discomfort."

The second list of self-statements should not be "written in stone." As one person told me, your initial production of that list allows you to format the approach. Once you begin to use the technique you can make adjustments as needed. Throw out statements that don't work and add new statements that do seem to be helpful.

In addition to replacing stressful thoughts, you also may want to release physical tension. There are a number of ways you can do this. One of the simplest is to take two deep breaths—the technique referred to in the impact phase of the example.

To use the deep breathing approach, begin by inhaling very slowly and deeply, then gradually exhale. Spend about two to three times as long exhaling as you do inhaling. After the first breath, take in a second deep breath and then let it out very slowly.

The only danger in this approach is hyperventilation—getting too much oxygen. To avoid this, simply imagine that you are holding a candle in front of your mouth and nose. Exhale only so as to flicker the flame of the candle but not so strongly as to blow it out.

Both the deep breathing approach and the stress inoculation training are intended to be used when your tension is fairly low, but you are expecting the pressure to increase. For instance, as the woman in the example, you may want to use your adaptive statements and take two deep breaths before you enter the hospital.

When you anticipate stressful circumstances, these techniques enable you to prepare effective strategies for dealing with the pressure. In a similar fashion, reading this book probably has been part of your preparation for helping a hospitalized patient. Having read the material, I hope you will feel more confident and competent as you offer support in a hospital setting.

Afterword

I asked visitors what they would like to accomplish the next time they see a hospitalized patient. Here are some typical responses.

- "I would hope that my visit would lift the spirits of the person I was visiting. I would bring to them anything I could to make them more comfortable or to help them entertain themselves during the times that they have no visitors. I would encourage the person to talk about anything he or she wanted to, for example, something that was bothering them or answer their questions about what was happening at home. I would also find out from that person what I could do to help his or her situation."
- "Basically, I would like to help [hospital patients] as much as I possibly can....I'd also like to just sit and listen. In my experiences, I can tell they like when someone just listens to them and lets them cry if they want; they feel very frustrated and confused and need a shoulder to cry on or someone to listen. Visits from friends seem extremely important because one friend once told me, 'When you're in the hospital, you find out who your friends truly are.'"
- "The next time I see a patient, I want to be able to be a good listener, [and I also want to be able to talk about topics other than the] present illness. My dad said he loved when we came to see him. It showed him how much we all care about and appreciate him. The experience definitely pulled my family together."

- "I [used to] hate visiting people but after being so critical and needing the support of friends and family to help me through the truamatic accident, [now] I don't mind."
- "I have been around a lot of deaths in my family and friends, and I have also been around close calls. I don't like to see people mangled or in pain, but I feel that if I were in that situation, I would want all the love and support I could get. Even if it is just sitting with the person and not talking, because I know it's uncomfortable talking when you're ill. I do not stay for long periods of time when I visit because I know that privacy and rest also are very important in recovery."
- "It brightens their day knowing that someone cares. A smile from a hospitalized patient is priceless."

How do you feel about seeing hospital patients, and what do you think of this book? I am interested in knowing your opinions. Your comments may help to improve subsequent editions of *The Hospital Patient*. If you would like to share your thoughts, write to me in care of New Day Publishers, P.O. Box 134, Carlisle, Pennsylvania 17013.

References

Chapter 1

Brodland, G. A., & Andreasen, N. J. C. (1977). Adjustment problems of the family of the burn patient. In R. H. Moos (Ed.), *Coping with physical illness* (pp. 167-176). New York: Plenum.

Chatham, M. A. (1978). The effect of family involvement on patients' manifestations of postcardiotomy psychosis. *Heart & Lung, 7*, 995-999.

Cobb, S., & Erbe, C. (1978). Social support for the cancer patient. *Forum on Medicine, 1* (8), 24-29.

Cotanch, P. H. (1984). Health promotion in hospitals. In J. D. Matarazzo, S. M. Weiss, J. A. Herd, N. E. Miller, & S. M. Weiss (Eds.), *Behavioral health: A handbook of health enhancement and disease prevention* (pp. 1125-1136). New York: Wiley.

Daley, L. (1984). The perceived immediate needs of families with relatives in the intensive care setting. *Heart & Lung, 13*, 231-237.

Dunkel-Schetter, C., & Wortman, C. (1982). The interpersonal dynamics of cancer: Problems in social relationships and their impact on the patient. In H. S. Friedman & M. R. DiMatteo (Eds.), *Interpersonal issues in health care* (pp. 69-100). New York: Academic Press.

Gore, S. (1985). Social support and styles of coping with stress. In S. Cohen and S. L. Syme, *Social support and health* (pp. 263-278). New York: Academic Press.

Hartsfield, J., & Clopton, J. R. (1985). Reducing presurgical anxiety: A possible visitor effect. *Social Science and Medicine, 20*, 529-533.

House, J. S., & Kahn, R. L. (1985). Measures and concepts of social suppport. In S. Cohen and S. L. Syme, *Social support and health* (pp. 83-108). New York: Academic Press.

Kerns, R. D., & Curley, A. D. (1985). A biopsychosocial approach to illness and the family: Neurological diseases across the life span. In D. C. Turk and R. D. Kerns (Eds.), *Health, illness, and families: A life-span perspective* (pp. 146-182). New York: Wiley.

Leventhal, H., Leventhal, E. A., & Nguyen, T. V. (1985). Reactions of families to illness: Theoretical models and perspectives. In D. C. Turk and R. D. Kerns (Eds.), *Health, illness, and families: A life-span perspective* (pp. 108-145). New York: Wiley.

Peters-Golden, H. (1982). Breast cancer: Varied perceptions of social support in the illness experience. *Social Science & Medicine, 16*, 483-491.

Porritt, D. (1979). Social support in crisis: Quantity or quality? *Social Science & Medicine, 13A*, 715-721.

Revenson, T. A., Wollman, C. A., & Felton, B. J. (1983). Social supports as stress buffers for adult cancer patients. *Psychosomatic Medicine, 45*, 321-331.

Sanders, G. S. (1982). Social comparison and perceptions of health and illness. In G. S. Sanders, & J. Suls (Eds.), *Social psychology of health and illness* (pp. 129-157). Hillsdale, NJ: Lawrence Erlbaum Associates.

Schulz, R., & Rau, M. T. (1985). Social support through the life course. In S. Cohen and S. L. Syme, *Social support and health* (pp. 129-149). New York: Academic Press.

Sosa, R., Kennell, J., Klaus, M., Robertson, S., & Urrutia, J. (1980). The effect of a supportive companion on perinatal problems, length of labor, and mother-infant interaction. *New England Journal of Medicine, 303*, 597-600.

Suls, J. (1982). Social support, interpersonal relations, and health: Benefits and liabilities. In G. S. Sanders, & J. Suls (Eds.), *Social psychology of health and illness* (pp. 255-277). Hillsdale, NJ: Lawrence Erlbaum Associates.

Turk, D. C., & Kerns, R. D. (1985). The family in health and illness. In D. C. Turk and R. D. Kerns (Eds.), *Health, illness, and families: A life-span perspective* (pp. 1-22). New York: Wiley.

Wills, T. A. (1985). Supportive fucntions of interpersonal relationships. In S. Cohen and S. L. Syme, *Social support and health* (pp. 61-82). New York: Academic Press.

Wortman, C. B. (1984). Social support and the cancer patient: Conceptual and methodologic issues. *Cancer, 53*, 2339-2360.

Wortman, C. B., & Conway, T. L. (1985). The role of social support in adaptation and recovery from physical illness. In S. Cohen and S. L. Syme, *Social support and health* (pp. 281-302). New York: Academic Press.

Chapter 2

Bulman, R.J., & Wortman, C.B. (1977). Attributions of blame and coping in the the "real world": Severe accident victims react to their lot. *Journal of Personality and Social Psychology, 35*, 351-363.

Cobb, S., & Erbe, C. (1978). Social support for the cancer patient. *Forum on Medicine, 1* (8), 24-29.

Nierenberg, J., & Janovic, F. (1985). *The hospital experience*. New York: Berkley Books.

Peters-Golden, H. (1982). Breast cancer: Varied perceptions of social support in the illness experience. *Social Science & Medicine, 16*, 483-491.

Porritt, D. (1979). Social support in crisis: Quantity or quality? *Social Science & Medicine, 13A*, 715-721.

Sanders, G. S. (1982). Social comparison and perceptions of health and illness. In G. S. Sanders, & J. Suls (Eds.), *Social psychology of health and illness* (pp. 129-157). Hillsdale, NJ: Lawrence Erlbaum Associates.

Suls, J. (1982). Social support, interpersonal relations, and health: Benefits and liabilities. In G. S. Sanders, & J. Suls (Eds.), *Social psychology of health and illness* (pp. 255-277). Hillsdale, NJ: Lawrence Erlbaum Associates.

Turk, D. C., & Kerns, R. D. (1985). The family in health and illness. In D. C. Turk and R. D. Kerns (Eds.), *Health, illness, and families: A life-span perspective* (pp. 1-22). New York: Wiley.

Wortman, C. B. (1984). Social support and the cancer patient: Conceptual and methodologic issues. *Cancer, 53*, 2339-2360.

Chapter 3

France, K. (1982). *Crisis intervention: A handbook of immediate person-to-person help.* Springfield, IL: Charles Thomas.

Lazarus, R. S. (1981). The costs and benefits of denial. In J. J. Spinetta and P. Deasy-Spinetta (Eds.), *Living with childhood cancer* (pp. 50-67). St. Louis: Mosby.

Vaughn, V. (1977). The vicissitudes and vivification of Viki Vaughn. In R. H. Moos (Ed.), *Coping with physical illness* (pp. 335-341). New York: Plenum.

Wortman, C. B. (1984). Social support and the cancer patient: Conceptual and methodologic issues. *Cancer, 53*, 2339-2360.

Wortman, C. B., & Lehman, D. R. (1985). Reactions to victims of life crises: Support attempts that fail. In I. G. Sarason & B. R. Sarason (Eds.), *Social support: Theory, research, and applications* (pp. 463-489). Boston: Martinus Hijhof.

Chapter 4

Dunkel-Schetter, C., & Wortman, C. (1982). The interpersonal dynamics of cancer: Problems in social relationships and their impact on the patient. In H. S. Friedman & M. R. DiMatteo (Eds.), *Interpersonal issues in health care* (pp. 69-100). New York: Academic Press.

Fordyce, W. E. (1976). *Behavioral methods for chronic pain and illness*. St. Louis: Mosby

Reimer, L. D., & Wagner, J. T. (1984). *The hospital handbook*. Wilton, CT: Morehouse Barlow.

Shipley, R. H., Butt, J. H., Horwitz, B. and Farbry, J. E. (1978). Preparation for a stressful medical procedure: Effect of amount of stimulus preexposure and coping style. *Journal of Consulting and Clinical Psychology, 46*, 499-507.

Whitcher, S. J., & Fisher, J. D. (1979). Multidimensional reaction to therapeutic touch in a hospital setting. *Journal of Personality and Social Psychology, 37*, 87-96.

Chapter 5

Alberti, R. E., & Emmons, M. L. (1982). *Your perfect right*. San Luis Obispo, CA: Impact Publishers.

Daley, L. (1984). The perceived immediate needs of families with relatives in the intensive care setting. *Heart & Lung, 13*, 231-237.

Dunkel-Schetter, C., & Wortman, C. (1982). The interpersonal dynamics of cancer: Problems in social relationships and their impact on the patient. In H. S. Friedman & M. R. DiMatteo (Eds.), *Interpersonal issues in health care* (pp. 69-100). New York: Academic Press.

Gots, R. E., & Kaufman, A. (1981). *People's hospital book*. New York: Avon.

Jones, M. L. (1985). *Home care for the chronically ill or disabled child*. New York: Harper & Row.

Nierenberg, J., & Janovic, F. (1985). *The hospital experience*. New York: Berkley Books.

Chapter 6

Adams-Greenly, M. (1986). Psychological staging of pediatric cancer patients and their families. *Cancer, 58*, 449-453.

Boyce, W. T. (1985). Social support, family relations, and children. In S. Cohen and S. L. Syme, *Social support and health* (pp. 151-173). New York: Academic Press.

Chatham, M. A. (1978). The effect of family involvement on patients' manifestations of postcardiotomy psychosis. *Heart & Lung, 7*, 995-999.

Gardner, D., & Stewart, N. (1978). Staff involvement with families of patients in critical-care units. *Heart & Lung, 7*, 105-110.

Heater, B. S. (1985). Nursing responsibilities in changing visiting restrictions in the intensive care unit. *Heart & Lung, 14*, 181-186.

Hoffman, I., & Futterman, E. H. (1977). Coping with waiting: Psychiatric intervention and study in the waiting room of a pediatric oncology clinic. In R. H. Moos (Ed.), *Coping with physical illness* (pp. 265-279). New York: Plenum.

Jones, M. L. (1985). *Home care for the chronically ill or disabled child.* New York: Harper & Row.

Kavanaugh, R. E. (1977). Humane treatment of the terminally ill. In R. H. Moos (Ed.), *Coping with physical illness* (pp. 413-419). New York: Plenum.

Kerns, R. D., & Curley, A. D. (1985). A biopsychosocial approach to illness and the family: Neurological diseases across the life span. In D. C. Turk and R. D. Kerns (Eds.), *Health, illness, and families: A life-span perspective* (pp. 146-182). New York: Wiley.

Kirchhoff, K. T. (1982). Visiting policies for patients with myocardial infarction: A national survey. *Heart & Lung, 11*, 571-576.

Klein, D. G. (1986). I.C.U.: It's also the intensive communication unit. *Nursing Life, 6* (1), 46-47.

Koocher, G. P. (1986). Psychosocial issues during the acute treatment of pediatric cancer. *Cancer, 58,* 468-472.

Mattsson, A. (1977). Long-term physical illness in childhood: A challenge to psychosocial adaptation. In R. H. Moos (Ed.), *Coping with physical illness* (pp. 183-199). New York: Plenum.

Melamed, B. G., & Bush, J. P. (1985). Family factors in children with acute illness. In D. C. Turk and R. D. Kerns (Eds.), *Health, illness, and families: A life-span perspective* (pp. 183-219). New York: Wiley.

Monaco, G. P. (1986). Resources available to the family of the child with cancer. *Cancer, 58,* 516-521.

Moos, R. H. (1977). The final crisis: Death and the fear of dying. In R. H. Moos (Ed.), *Coping with physical illness* (pp. 397-401). New York: Plenum.

Myers, B. A., Friedman, S. B., & Weiner, I. B. (1977). Coping with a chronic disability: Psychosocial observations of girls with scoliosis. In R. H. Moos (Ed.), *Coping with physical illness* (pp. 219-232). New York: Plenum.

Rothstein, P. (1980). Psychological stress in families of children in a pediatric intensive care unit. *Pediatric Clinics of North America, 27,* 613-620.

Stillwell, S. B. (1984). Importance of visiting needs as perceived by family members of patients in the intensive care unit. *Heart & Lung, 13,* 238-242.

Youngner, S. J., Coulton, C., Welton, R., Juknialis, B., Jackson, D. L. (1984). ICU visiting policies. *Critical Care Medicine, 12,* 606-608.

Chapter 7

Adams-Greenly, M. (1986). Psychological staging of pediatric cancer patients and their families. *Cancer, 58,* 449-453.

Baranowski, T., & Nader, P. R. (1985). Family health behavior. In D. C. Turk and R. D. Kerns (Eds.), *Health, illness, and families: A life-span perspective*

(pp. 51-80). New York: Wiley.
Bedsworth, J. A. & Molen, M. T. (1982). Psychological stress in spouses of patients with myocardial infarction. *Heart & Lung, 11*, 450-456.
Bordow, S., & Porritt, D. (1979). An experimental evaluation of crisis intervention. *Social Science and Medicine, 13A*, 251-256.
Capone, M. A., Good, R. S., Westie, K. S., & Jacobson, A. F. (1980). Psychosocial rehabilitation of gynecologic oncology patients. *Archives of Physical Medicine and Rehabilitation, 61*, 128-132.
Capone, M. A., Westie, K. S., Chitwood, J. S., Feigenbaum, D., & Good, R. S. (1979). Crisis intervention: A functional model for hospitalized cancer patients. *American Journal of Orthopsychiatry, 49*, 598-607.
Cobb, S., & Erbe, C. (1978). Social support for the cancer patient. *Forum on Medicine, 1* (8), 24-29.
D'Afflitti, J. G., & Weitz, G. W. (1977). Rehabilitating the stroke patient through patient-family groups. In R. H. Moos (Ed.), *Coping with physical illness* (pp. 135-144). New York: Plenum.
Dunkel-Schetter, C., & Wortman, C. (1982). The interpersonal dynamics of cancer: Problems in social relationships and their impact on the patient. In H. S. Friedman & M. R. DiMatteo (Eds.), *Interpersonal issues in health care* (pp. 69-100). New York: Academic Press.
France, K. (1982). *Crisis intervention: A handbook of immediate person-to-person help*. Springfield, IL: Charles Thomas.
Gruen, W. (1975). Effects of brief psychotherapy during the hospitalization period on the recovery process in heart attacks. *Journal of Consulting and Clinical Psychology, 43*, 223-232.
Hodovanic, B. H., Reardon, D., Reese, W., & Hedges, B. (1984). Family crisis intervention program in the medical intensive care unit. *Heart & Lung, 13*, 243-249.

Johnson. S. B. (1985). The family and the child with chronic illness. In D. C. Turk and R. D. Kerns (Eds.), *Health, illness, and families: A life-span perspective* (pp. 220-254). New York: Wiley.

Kaplan, D. M., Smith, A., Grobstein, R., and Fischman, S. E. (1977). Family mediation of stress. In R. H. Moos (Ed.), *Coping with physical illness* (pp. 81-96). New York: Plenum.

Knafl, K. A., Deatrick, J. A., & Kodadek, S. (1982). How parents manage jobs and a child's hospitalization. *American Journal of Maternal Child Nursing, 7* (March/April), 125-127.

Koocher, G. P. (1986). Psychosocial issues during the acute treatment of pediatric cancer. *Cancer, 58,* 468-472.

Meichenbaum, D. (1977). *Cognitive-behavior modification: An integrative approach.* New York: Plenum.

Meichenbaum, D. (1985). *Stress inoculation training.* New York: Pergamon.

Monaco, G. P. (1986). Resources available to the family of the child with cancer. *Cancer, 58,* 516-521.

Mumford, E., Schlesinger, H. J., & Glass, G. V. (1982). The effects of psychological intervention on recovery from surgery and heart attacks: An analysis of the literature. *American Journal of Public Health, 72,* 141-151.

Porritt, D. (1979). Social support in crisis: Quantity or quality? *Social Science & Medicine, 13A,* 715-721.

Rothstein, P. (1980). Psychological stress in families of children in a pediatric intensive care unit. *Pediatric Clinics of North America, 27,* 613-620.

Tropauer, A., Franz, M. N., & Dilgard, V. W. (1977). Psychological aspects of the care of children with cystic fibrosis. In R. H. Moos (Ed.), *Coping with physical illness* (pp. 201-218). New York: Plenum.

Wortman, C. B. (1984). Social support and the cancer patient: Conceptual and methodologic issues. *Cancer, 53,* 2339-2360.

Index

Action figures, 92
Advice
　intent and risks of, 49-51
　medical, 10
Advocate
　and decision making, 29-31
　interactions with staff, 83-85
　long visits by, 31, 71
Aides, 80, 81
Allergic reaction, 9
Alphabet board, 106
Analysis, 47-49
Appendectomy, 17
Art supplies, 92
Assertive communication, 86-88
Attendants, 80, 81
Attending physician
　change in, 79-80
　responsibilities, 76-77, 82, 121
　sleep - over support from, 95
Auto accident, 8, 14, 19

Bathing, 13, 90-91

Books, 11
Boredom, 28
Brain death, 119
Brain injury patients
　social isolation of, 2
　visitor guidelines, 110-112

Canada, 95
Cancer patients, 2, 22, 23, 49, 67
Cassette player/recorder
　for a child, 93
　popular gift, 12
Cassette tapes, 12, 63, 93
Cerebrovascular accident.
　See Stroke
Charge nurse
　responsibilities, 81
　ICU, 108
Chatham, Margaret Ann, 106-107
Child care, 14, 15
Children, 90-103
　brothers and sisters of, 102-103
　concerns of, 91-93, 99
　distortion to, 94

ending visits with, 94-95
objects and, 91-92
length of visits to, 98
nonjudgmental with, 94,
 100-102
perceptiveness of, 99-100
permanence and, 90
preparing yourself for, 94
rooming-in with, 95-97
self-care of, 90-91
visits by, 63-64, 108
wondering about
 symptoms, 98
Church, 7
Christmas shopping, 14
Coma, 106, 119, 133
Common sense
 during visitor crises, 137
 using this book, 5
 while being an advocate,
  30
Construction toys, 92
Coronary bypass, 106-107
Craft kits, 92
Crises, 125-142
 patient, 125-128
 patient coping, 135
 visitor, 128-135
 visitor coping, 135-142
CVA. See Stroke

Death
 informing accident victim,
  8
 thinking about, 99,
  113-116
 survivor reactions to,
  121-122
Decision making, 23-31
 and children, 96, 101

and ICU discharge, 109
and patients in crisis, 135
and treatment termination,
 119-121
and visitors in crisis,
 137-138
steps in
 alternatives, 24-25
 plan, 25-26
 thoughts and feelings,
  24
typical concerns, 27-29
Delusions, 104, 107, 132
Denial
 of children's concerns, 94
 as an initial reaction, 129
 in response to reflection,
  41
Depression
 in brain injury patients,
  111
 in children, 99
 limit reflection of, 42-43
Director of nursing, 82
Dolls, 92
Durable power of attorney,
 120

Empathy, 22-23, 39
Errands
 for patient, 14
 for patient's parents, 102
 for patient's spouse, 15
Etiquette
 deciding how long to stay,
  70-72
 demonstrating respect,
  64-70
 planning, 57-64

Flowers
  caring for, 13
  not ICU gifts, 108
Folk medicine, 9
Food
  gifts of, 11
  not ICU gifts, 108

Games
  as focus of visit, 91
  as gifts, 11
Gifts
  ease of giving, 31
  for children, 91-92
  possibilities, 10-12
Guidance, 9

Hair washing, 13
Hallucinations, 104
Head nurse, 81
Home remedies, 9
Honesty
  assertiveness and, 87
  encouraged, 31
  positive relationship and, 21
  reflection and, 40
  terminal patients and, 117-119
  visitor crises and, 137
Household responsibilities
  of patient, 8, 14
  of patient's parents, 102
  of patient's spouse, 15
  of visitors, 134
Humor, 16-18

ICU. *See* Intensive care unit patients

ICU psychosis, 104
Information, 7-10
  about the outside, 7-8
  ease of giving, 31
  need for, 82-83
  pain reduction and, 61
Interns, 78
Interrogation, 35-38
  appropriateness, 38
  closed questions, 36-37, 53
  open-ended questions, 35-36
  questions to avoid, 53-55
  sequences of, 37-38
  See also Questions
Introducing yourself, 66
Intensive care unit patients, 103-109
  ICU psychosis, 104
  physical setting, 103-104
  transfer from unit, 108-109
  unit staff, 103
  visiting guidelines, 105-107
  visitor restrictions, 107-108
Isolation, 28, 126

Joking
  do's and don'ts of, 16-18
  suitable for you, 31

Knocking, 65

Length of visit
  common concern, 29
  guidelines for, 70-72

with children, 98
with ICU patients, 108
with psychiatric patients,
   110
Licensed practical nurse, 80,
   81
Living will, 120

Mail, 14
Massachusetts, 95
Magazine, 11
Mealtime, 13
Medical advice, 9-10
Medical chart, 76-77
Medical information, 9
Medical personnel. *See* Staff
Meichenbaum, Donald,
   138-139
Moral support
   guidelines for, 15-23
      discussing pleasant
         times, 16
      joking and kidding,
         16-18
      prayer and scripture,
         18-19
      positive relationship
         and, 20-23
      responding to
         uncertainty, 19-20,
         21
   following ICU discharge,
      109
   for children, 96
   for patients in crisis, 135
   for visitors in crisis,
      137-138
   suitable for you, 31
Morale, 15

Myasthenia gravis, 23

News events, 7, 105
Newspaper, 11
Note pad, 53
Nursing coordinator, 81
Nursing staff
   description, 80-82
   ICU, 103
   See also Staff
Nurses' station
   confrontation cite, 86
   first stop, 64
   information depository, 95
   information source, 62, 65
   psychiatric units, 110
   source of help, 84

Orderlies, 80, 81
Overindulgence, 101-102
Overprotectiveness
   of clearheaded patients,
      23-24
   leading to humiliation, 50

Pain
   analyzed, 47-48
   do's and don'ts, 59-62
   evaluating in children, 97
Pets
   checking on, 14
   information about, 8
   visits by, 91
Physician specialities, 77-78
Physicians. *See* Staff
Pity, 46
Playroom, 91
Political topics, 7
Positive relationship

components of, 20-23
reflection and, 40
Prayer
  suggestions for, 18-19
  suitable for you, 31
Primary care nurse
  responsibilities, 81
  ICU, 103
Privacy, 65
Problem solving, 24-26
  See also Decision making
Prognosis
  defined, 82
  of children, 99
  of ICU patients, 108
  of terminal patients, 116-117
  poor, 20
Psychiatric patients, 109-110
Puppets, 92
Puzzles
  as focus of visit, 91
  popular gift, 11

Questions
  appropriateness, 38
  children afraid to ask, 92-93
  closed, 36-37, 53, 112
  from patient, 82
  from children, 98
  leading, 54
  multiple, 53-54, 112
  obtaining medical information, 8, 85
  open-ended, 35-36
  problem solving and, 24
  sequences of, 37-38
  to brain injury patients, 112
  to children, 97
  to ICU patients, 106
  to reticent patients, 43-45
  to staff, 69, 83
  "why," 54-55, 87

Reading, 13, 93
Reassurance, 52
Reflection, 39-45
  definition, 39
  emotional intensity of, 41-42
  of staff responses, 88
  positive relationship and, 22
  problem solving and, 24, 85, 93
Registered nurses, 80, 81
Relaxation, 142
Resident physicians, 78
Respect
  encouraged, 31
  postive relationship and, 21-22
  ways to demonstrate, 27, 64-70
Ronald McDonald House, 97
Rooming-in, 95-97
Roommate, 28-29

School
  as conversation topic, 7, 91
  assignments, 100
Scripture

source of comfort, 18
suitable for you, 31
Self-blame
  by patients, 22
  by visitors, 101-102, 130
Self-care in children, 90-91, 101
Self-control, 62
Self-deception, 41
Self-disclosure
  and children, 100
  encouraging, 27
Self-doubt, 21, 115-116
Self-esteem, 15, 21, 127
Self-statements, 139-142
Self-worth, 23
Service clubs, 7
Shifts, 81
Sitting, 67
Sleep
  awaken from or not, 65-66
  etiquette and, 59
  pain increase and, 48, 61
Sleep-over, 95-97
Smoking, 64
Social comparison, 19
Soap opera, 8
Social service department
  source of information, 97
  visitor support from, 137-138
Special care unit
  advocate responsibility and, 30
  ICU, 103-109
Sports, 7, 105
Staff
  dissatisfaction with, 27-28, 69-70, 75-76, 119
  interacting with, 82-88
  interns, 78
  not butt of jokes, 16
  nursing staff, 80-82
    charge nurse, 81, 108
    director of nursing, 82
    head nurse, 81
    licensed practical nurses, 80, 81
    primary care nurse, 30, 81, 103
    registered nurses, 80, 81
    vocational nurses, 81
  other staff members, 82
  physicians
    attending physician, 76-77, 79-80, 82, 95, 121
    medical specialties, 77-78
    residents, 78
  satisfaction with, 28, 74-75
  trust in, 69
  when to ask questions of, 69, 83
Stress inoculation training, 138-142
Stress management, 138-142
Stroke, 111
Stroke patients, 110-112
Stuffed animals, 90, 92
Suicidal teenagers, 43-45
Support groups, 138
Surgery
  advocate responsibility

and, 30-31, 98, 120
presurgery food
restrictions, 9
priorities after, 31, 57,
106-107
touch after, 68, 107
Sympathy, 46

Tasks for patients
and degree of intimacy, 31
inside the hospital, 13-14
outside the hospital,
14-15
with terminal patients,
118
Telephone call, 62-63
Terminal patients, 112-121
decision-making support
and, 117-119
ending treatment of,
119-121
learning of a terminal
diagnosis, 116-117
thinking about death,
113-116
Terminal diagnosis, 116-117

Touch
children and, 93
guidelines for, 67-68
ICU patients and, 107
terminal patients and, 117
Toy, 90, 91-92
Traumatic brain injury, 111

Uncertainty, 19-20, 21
Unconscious, 8, 29
Understanding
encouraged, 31
positive relationship and,
22
ways of demonstrating,
39-45

Vocational nurse, 81

Weather, 7, 105
Work, 7
Writing
by ICU patients, 106
instead of visiting, 63
materials, 12, 92
when communication is
difficult, 53, 112

Order Form

New Day Publishers
Department B
P.O. Box 134
Carlisle, PA 17013

Please send me _____ copies of

The Hospital Patient
A Guide for Family and Friends

___ copies x $9.95 =   _____

Shipping (choose one)
Book rate (4 weeks): add
$1.25 for first book and 25¢
for each additional book

or

Air mail: add $3.00 per book   _____

Pennsylvania residents add
60¢ sales tax for each book   _____

Amount enclosed =   _____

Name: _____

Address:_____

_____

Zip: _____

Order Form

New Day Publishers
Department B
P.O. Box 134
Carlisle, PA 17013

Please send me _____ copies of
The Hospital Patient
A Guide for Family and Friends

___ copies x $9.95 = _____

Shipping (choose one)
Book rate (4 weeks): add
$1.25 for first book and 25¢
for each additional book

       or

Air mail: add $3.00 per book _____

Pennsylvania residents add
60¢ sales tax for each book _____

Amount enclosed = _____

Name: _____

Address:_____

       _____

       Zip: _____

Order Form

New Day Publishers
Department B
P.O. Box 134
Carlisle, PA 17013

Please send me _____ copies of
The Hospital Patient
A Guide for Family and Friends

___ copies x $9.95 =   _____

Shipping (choose one)
Book rate (4 weeks): add
$1.25 for first book and 25¢
for each additional book

        or

Air mail: add $3.00 per book   _____

Pennsylvania residents add
60¢ sales tax for each book   _____

Amount enclosed =   _____

Name: _____

Address: _____

_____

    Zip: _____